We Are One In Eight

18 real stories of infertility, IVF, loss and hope

For Eoin,
the bravest little superman.

Forever in our hearts
and always by Lucia's side.

Contents

On average, around the world:

1 in 8
experience fertility problems

1 in 4
pregnancies ends in miscarriage

1 in 80
pregnancies are ectopic

Foreword

One in eight experience fertility problems, yet it's still deemed a taboo subject. Many women and couples feel as though fertility treatments are something they have to hide from people, even those closest to them. An infertility diagnosis can be overwhelming, emotional, expensive, strain your relationships, and cause feelings of stress, anxiety and inadequacy. Anyone can be affected – infertility does not discriminate.

By sharing our stories, we hope to raise awareness, break down stigmas and let others know that they're not alone. There is a community who can help support you, offer comfort, and give hope where needed. We hope that people reading this will recognise parts of themselves and their situations in our experiences and feel seen. There are many different causes of infertility, treatment options and outcomes, but one thing the women in this book have in common (no matter what stage we're at currently), is that the communities we've found during our journeys have helped us in so many ways – inspiring, educating and supporting us through some of the most difficult times of our lives. Reach out to us; to the infertility, trying to conceive and IVF communities (among others), and know that you aren't alone.

From the other perspective, if you know someone who's having a hard time trying to conceive, going through IVF, grieving the loss of a baby, or making the difficult decision to stop treatment, these journeys might give a little more insight into ways to better support and understand them.

These stories are raw, emotional and sometimes difficult to read. Certain parts may be triggering (depending on your own experience), so we've included a small overview at the start of each, highlighting some of the aspects talked about.

Each of the women/couples have also chosen a charity to donate a portion of our proceeds to, with a full list at the end of the book. We hope that we can help support these important charities, as well as supporting others in this community.

So, to all those navigating through infertility: We see you. We are you. We are one in eight.

Glossary of terms

The world of infertility and trying to conceive is a minefield of acronyms and abbreviations. We've put together a handy list of some of the main terms, to help when reading this book or to refer back to during your own journey.

AMH – Anti-Mullerian Hormone *(this level indicates your ovarian egg reserve)*
ART – Assisted Reproductive Technology
AH – Assisted Hatching *(procedure allowing a fertilised embryo to 'hatch')*
BAME – Black, Asian and minority ethnic
BBT – Basal body temperature
Beta – Blood test to check your HCG levels
BFP – Big fat positive *(positive pregnancy test)*
BFN – Big fat negative *(negative pregnancy test)*
BIPOC – Black, Indigenous and people of colour
Blastocyst – early stage of an embryo *(5 days after fertilisation)*
CCG – Clinical Commissioning Group *(responsible for planning and commissioning health care services in local areas)*
DC – Donor conception
D&C – Dilation and curettage *(a procedure to remove tissue from inside your uterus, also used after a miscarriage)*
DCDA – Dichorionic Diamniotic twins *(each baby has a separate placenta and amniotic sac)*
DEIVF – Donor egg IVF
Down regulation – 'Switching off' your ovaries with fertility drugs
DPT – Days post transfer *(e.g. 3dp5dt is 3 days post 5-day transfer)*
DSIVF – Donor sperm IVF
Endo– Endometriosis
EPAU/EPU – Early Pregnancy (Assessment) Unit
ERA – Endometrial Receptivity Analysis *(a test to determine the best day to transfer an embryo during an IVF cycle)*
FET – Frozen embryo transfer *(more info in the outline of treatments)*

FSH – Follicle-Stimulating Hormone *(regulates your menstrual cycle)*

HCG – Human Chorionic Gonadotropin *(the pregnancy hormone that blood and urine tests detect)*

HSG – Hysterosalpingogram *(procedure to investigate the shape of the uterine cavity and patency of the fallopian tubes)*

ICSI – Intracytoplasmic sperm injection *(more info in the outline of treatments)*

Implantation – When an embryo attaches to the wall of your uterus

IUI – Intrauterine Insemination *(more info in the outline of treatments)*

IVF – In vitro fertilisation *(more info in the outline of treatments)*

LH – Luteinising Hormone *(regulates the function of your ovaries or testes)*

LP – Luteal Phase *(part of your menstrual cycle where uterus lining thickens after ovulation)*

MCDA – Monochorionic Diamniotic twins *(the babies share a placenta but have separate amniotic sacs)*

MCMA – Monochorionic Monoamniotic twins *(the babies share a placenta and amniotic sac)*

MFI – Male factor infertility

NICE – National Institute for Health and Care Excellence

NICU – Neonatal Intensive Care Unit

OB/OBGYN – Obstetrician or Obstetrician-Gynaecologist

OHSS – Ovarian Hyperstimulation Syndrome

OPK – Ovulation predictor kit

OTD – Official test day *(date given to take a pregnancy test after transfer)*

PAL – Pregnancy after loss

PCOS – Polycystic Ovary Syndrome

PGS – Pre-implantation genetic screening *(having the chromosomes of embryos checked for abnormalities before transfer)*
PIO – Progesterone in Oil injection
PND – Postnatal depression
POAS – Pee on a stick *(take a pregnancy test)*
POC – People of colour
PTSD – Post-traumatic stress disorder
PUPO – Pregnant until proven otherwise
Pulling the 'trigger' – The injection you take to release your eggs *(36 hours before your egg collection)*
RE – Reproductive Endocrinologist
RIVF – Reciprocal IVF
RPL – Recurrent pregnancy loss
Scanxiety – Anxiety at each scan throughout pregnancy
SCBU – Special Care Baby Unit
SIS – Saline infusion sonohysterography *(a procedure to evaluate the uterus and the shape of the uterine cavity)*
SMBC – Single mother by choice
Stims – Stimulation phase of hormone injections
TS – Traditional surrogacy
TSH – Thyroid-stimulating hormone *(you can have a test to measure how much of this hormone is in your blood)*
TTC – Trying to conceive
TTTS – Twin to twin transfusion syndrome
TWW – Two-week wait *(time between transfer/ovulation and your test day/expected period)*
Wanda – Vaginal ultrasound probe *(nickname from the TTC community)*

Outline of treatments

Every journey is different, and protocols and medications vary from person to person, but here's a brief overview of the main fertility treatments you may encounter while trying to conceive, which are also detailed throughout the stories in this book.

Fertility drugs

Fertility drugs, most commonly Clomifene Citrate (Clomid®), can be used in the treatment of some women who've been trying to get pregnant but have been unable to do so naturally. They're the main treatment for women who have fertility issues related to Polycystic Ovary Syndrome, and men and women who have fertility issues related to hormone imbalances.

IUI (Intrauterine Insemination)

IUI, also known as artificial insemination, is a type of fertility treatment in which the better-quality sperm are separated from sperm that are sluggish, non-moving or abnormally shaped. These sperm are then injected directly into the womb around the time of ovulation. IUI may be performed with a partner's sperm or donor sperm (known as donor insemination).

IVF (In vitro fertilisation)

IVF is a type of fertility treatment where fertilisation takes place outside the body. The woman takes fertility hormones to stimulate her ovaries to produce multiple eggs. These eggs are then collected in a retrieval procedure and mixed with sperm in a laboratory. IVF is carried out when the sperm quality is considered to be 'normal'. If there are any issues, such as low motility or numbers, a procedure called ICSI (see below) will be used instead.

If fertilisation is successful, the embryos are allowed to develop for between two and six days. This helps the embryologist select the strongest embryo, which is then transferred back to the woman's womb, to hopefully continue to a successful pregnancy and birth.

If several good quality embryos are created, these can be frozen to use at a later date (see FET below).

ICSI (Intracytoplasmic sperm injection)

For around half of couples who are having problems conceiving, the cause of infertility is sperm-related. ICSI is a common and successful treatment for male infertility. It may be recommended if you have low sperm count, poor motility or poor morphology (abnormal shape), or if you have previously had IVF but very few, or none, of the eggs fertilised. It's performed as part of IVF and involves selected sperm being injected directly into the egg.

FET (Frozen embryo transfer)

If you have IVF or ICSI and have good quality embryos left after transfer, or if you had a freeze-all cycle, these can be frozen to use in the future (for example if your first transfer is unsuccessful or if you want to try for another baby). Frozen embryos are thawed and transferred into the womb after suitable preparation of the womb lining.

An FET cycle is gentler on your body, as it doesn't involve stimulation of your ovaries or an egg collection. The majority involve hormone regulation, with oestrogen and progesterone, although in some cases it's possible to have a natural cycle. Although most embryos survive the thawing process, there is a small risk that some may not.

Lauren and Rich

After four years of trying to conceive and four treatment cycles (IUI, IVF and two FETs), they had twins in July 2020. They talk about their experience with male factor infertility, using a sperm donor, failed cycles and pregnancy after IVF.

Lauren

After six years together, Rich and I got married in August 2015. I'd just turned 30, Rich was 31 and we had a house and a dog, so we decided it was the 'right' time to start expanding our family. Like many others, we started a bit naively, thinking I'd just fall pregnant within a few months – after all, I'd spent so many years on birth control trying not to get pregnant!

It began quite casually, not 'really trying', and we were busy with work and life. We live in Kent, England and I work as a graphic designer and Rich is a nurse, specialising in cardiology. We had holidays and social events booked so there was no pressure. However, after about six months of nothing happening, we started tracking my ovulation using fertility apps and ovulation tests. I began eating a bit healthier and taking the right vitamins. Trying to conceive (TTC) is an expensive business – I took Pregnacare® for years and bought dozens of ovulation kits and pregnancy tests. Each month became a waiting game to see if I was pregnant, then the disappointment that I wasn't, then waiting for the next ovulation, the next pregnancy test, and on and on.

A few people close to us announced pregnancies during that first year. My sister and sister-in-law fell pregnant, a couple of friends and work colleagues, and at the beginning it didn't affect me too much. We were trying too so I would excitedly think, 'it'll be us next' but as time went on, it became more painful. Would it be us next? Why was nothing happening? People would ask when we were having kids, and it became harder to brush it off with an 'oh, maybe next year' or 'hopefully soon'. I began to dread being asked.

I didn't realise at the start how much waiting TTC would involve. After just over a year of unsuccessful trying, I went to see the GP. Following some investigation for extremely painful periods as a teenager, I'd been diagnosed with mild polycystic ovary syndrome (PCOS), and in my early twenties I'd had a couple of colposcopy laser treatments to remove abnormal cells from my cervix (ladies, please have your smear tests). I figured those might be reasons why we weren't falling pregnant so the doctor referred me to the local hospital for some investigation.

While waiting for the hospital appointments, 2017 became the worst year of our lives. In the April, one of our closest friends, Chris, was diagnosed with stage 4 bowel cancer. He fought hard for five months, but the cancer had spread too far and he sadly died in the September, when his baby daughter was only seven months old.

During that heartbreaking time, TTC wasn't at the forefront of our minds. I had a couple of hospital appointments over those months and they couldn't see any obvious factors that were affecting my fertility – my ovaries were even deemed to be fine, so my diagnosis of mild PCOS when I was younger may have been incorrect. They then asked Rich to give a sperm sample to try and rule out any issues there.

We had our last hospital appointment in October 2017, the day after Chris' funeral. I remember us sitting in the waiting room, still devastated and numb from the day before. The doctor told us that we'd need to be referred to Kings fertility clinic in London, as Rich's sample had come back with no sperm present. The technical term is azoospermia. We were shocked to hear there was no sperm at all, at worst we'd thought maybe just a low count or low motility.

We then had another three-month wait for our first fertility clinic appointment. By this time, we'd been trying for two years and had no idea when or how we might be able to conceive. The clinic conducted a repeat of all the tests we'd had at the hospital and came to the same conclusions: no sperm present, no visible other factors. Fertility clinics are specialists when it comes to female fertility issues and have numerous gynaecologists, however they don't have any male specialists, so we would once again need to be referred – this time to a urologist, who could see if Rich had a reason for the infertility, such as a blockage.

We'd assumed a urologist was the only specialist for male fertility after being referred there by the clinic, however after watching a Rhod Gilbert documentary on male factor infertility (MFI) recently, we found out there are actually other male specialists called andrologists, who may have been able to offer some extra advice.

The urologist we were referred to was one of the leading ones in the country, however that unfortunately meant there was a nine-month waiting list to see him – crushingly the same length as a pregnancy. I called every week in the hope of getting a cancellation appointment but they never had any, so it felt like everything was on hold. There was no chance we could get pregnant naturally, so each month it felt more and more like we were wasting time, and eggs.

I asked the clinic about possibly collecting and freezing my eggs during that long wait, but they assured me that with my age and good AMH number then my egg reserve should be fine. They also told us at the time that it was better for us to freeze embryos rather than eggs.

Inevitably during that long period of time, more people around us fell pregnant. The emotional toll of trying for a baby is one I wasn't fully prepared for. I absolutely love my friends and family, and was of course happy and excited for them when they announced pregnancies, but there was always a part of me that was sad for us. When would it be our turn? I still look at children who were conceived when we started trying and wonder what life would be like if we had a 4-year old running around with them. We might've been trying for a sibling now.

I went to baby showers, to visit newborns and to children's birthday parties during those years, and I don't mind admitting that it was tough. There were days when I thought, 'If one more person tells me they're pregnant, I'm going to break'. It is ok not to be ok all of the time. It doesn't mean I don't love all the children in my life and am happy for other people, it's just hard.

I began to run a lot more during that time as a physical outlet for my emotions and built up the distance until I signed up to run a marathon. I also occupied my time outside of work with helping to set up a charity with Chris' wife, Kirsty, and some friends: The Chris Aked Foundation. We support children of families who are dealing with cancer and other life-affecting illnesses, offering help through memory-making days, activities and counselling. I threw myself into writing as well and kept permanently busy, although TTC was always at the surface of my mind. It's hard not to let it take over your life.

We eventually got our urology appointment in September 2018. The urologist was great, but there was never much interest in finding a specific cause for the infertility, only potential treatments. They think it may have stemmed from a serious illness Rich had in his late teens that could affect sperm production, although he also had low testosterone, which may have been a factor. They couldn't find any obvious blockages from their initial investigation.

Something we learnt, is that any long-term treatment to increase testosterone ironically causes temporary infertility. Similar to steroids, it decreases sperm production by decreasing the FSH hormone, so it was advised that hormone treatment for increasing Rich's testosterone permanently wouldn't start until after we'd tried options to conceive.

Before any invasive surgery, the first treatment we were offered was a three-month course of Clomid® (Clomiphene citrate) for Rich. This wasn't fully approved for men at the time, so more of a trial treatment to see if it improved sperm count. It was better than immediate surgery though, so we tried the course at the end of 2018 – a whole year that had been lost waiting for a referral, and now three years after we began trying.

For those three months, it felt like there was a glimmer of hope again with trying naturally, and I found myself symptom spotting during the two-week wait, even though I knew the chances were slim. We had a holiday to Antigua during that time, a break that we both needed but still something that played on my mind with TTC. The country had a higher Zika virus level than other places, what if I got pregnant there and contracted Zika? You're advised not to have fertility treatment for three months after visiting a place with a high level just in case. That was something I never thought we'd be worrying about, but now everything came into question. We knew our odds were miniscule, although it still didn't stop me being extra careful of bites.

Unfortunately, the Clomid® didn't improve any sperm

count, so then it was on to the next part: a micro-TESE – a surgery that involves going into the testicle to see if sperm can be removed from the tubes inside.

It would be invasive, painful surgery and I didn't want to pressure Rich into having it, but he'd decided to pursue every avenue in order to possibly have biological children, so there wouldn't be any questions of 'what if' later. By that point, we'd had a couple of brief discussions about the idea of using a sperm donor, but were still hopeful it wouldn't come to that.

The operation was booked for April 2019 (two days after I ran the marathon so we were a sight both hobbling out of the clinic afterwards!). The surgery itself ended up being a double micro-TESE, as the clinic wanted to make sure they'd tried everything they could, but that made the recovery twice as painful. While Rich was still under the anaesthetic, the doctor came to tell me that unfortunately they hadn't been able to retrieve any sperm to use. When Rich came round, I felt awful having to break the news to him. It was devastating to know the surgery had been unsuccessful and that we'd never have any chance of conceiving naturally or having a child that was biologically ours.

We took some time to process the news, then had a decision to make. At the start, the thought of using a sperm donor seemed overwhelming, but the more we researched, the less scary it became. We found lots of information on the HFEA (Human Fertilisation & Embryology Authority) and Donor Conception Network websites.

There were a lot of questions: How would we find a donor? How much would it cost? How did it work with telling a possible future child they were donor conceived? Would they be able to find their donor when they were older?

Our clinic had mandatory counselling for anyone considering donor conception, to talk through questions and make sure you were ready to proceed with treatment. Not being able to have your own child is a loss and you need time to process your emotions and to grieve. Unfortunately with our situation, we'd had a year-long wait to think things through. Of course, we'd hoped more than anything that the Clomid® or surgery might have had a good outcome, but we'd also mentally prepared for the worst.

It was more difficult for Rich to come to terms with though; there would be no baby that was biologically his. I think it's harder for men mentally, as there's nowhere near the level of support out there as there is for women. You can find thousands of Instagram accounts and social media support groups for women, but hardly any for men.

We had also discussed the idea of adoption – something that's close to our family, as Rich's parents are foster carers and we've seen a lot of children go through the adoption process over the years. I wanted to hopefully experience pregnancy so we decided to first try for a child that would be biologically mine with donor sperm.

The counselling session was informative and we learnt the law had changed in the UK in 1991 to mean that any donor-conceived child can find out who their donor is when they turn 18 years old. That meant any donor we chose would need to be non-anonymous, so our potential child would be able to find them in the future. We wouldn't know who they were, unless our child wanted to find out. Each donor has a legal limit of how many families they can donate to (pregnancy quota), although you can pay to have donor exclusivity.

We found out there are lots of books and resources for talking to a child in the future about their conception. It's recommended that you begin to tell them at a young age, so their story becomes a normal part of life, rather than a big secret they might be shocked to find out as an older child or even an adult. That can lead to emotional issues or them lashing out as they struggle to understand their conception.

At this stage, it was all a hypothetical situation of us having had a child – we hadn't even chosen the donor, let alone started the treatment process yet. The counsellor signed off on us being ready to proceed so the next step was a treatment plan. The treatment you're allowed as part of the NHS varies depending on your postcode and situation. Some places offer one, two or three IVF cycles, some don't offer any, so it's a bit of a lottery!

The NICE guidelines state that women under 40 should be offered three full cycles of IVF (which is one egg collection and then transfer of any resultant fresh and frozen embryos), however local hospitals are governed by the Clinical Commissioning Group (CCG), who set their own rules per area. As Rich and I met the right criteria for our area (we didn't have any children, were the right BMI and age, and had been trying for over two years) we were eligible to have some treatment funded by the NHS.

We were offered three IUIs and one full IVF cycle. One cycle. Not three. It was also capped at three embryo transfers for us, regardless of how many embryos we got. We had no real knowledge of IVF and had no idea how the process would work, or if we would even get enough embryos to freeze to have three transfer attempts (it's no guarantee) so it felt like there was a lot of pressure on this one round.

The IUI procedure is much less invasive so we chose to try that treatment first, and the next hurdle was finding a sperm donor. It was now mid-May 2019 and it felt like things were finally moving at a much quicker pace after so many years of waiting. The clinic gave us a list of a few UK and international sperm banks they used so we could find our donor.

We started off looking at a couple of UK sperm banks, knowing they would all comply with non-anonymous donors. We wanted to find a donor who would be similar to Rich in terms of looks and build. The UK banks we searched seemed very light on available donors though, and once we'd narrowed down a few criteria, we were left with only three potential matches. Reading the profiles, we weren't drawn to any of them.

We then decided to try Cryos International bank in Denmark – one of the biggest sperm banks in the world. Compared to the UK ones, it was surprising how much you could input for your search and how much detail they gave you on the profiles. After selecting our preferred criteria, and choosing non-anonymous donors, we were left with nearly 100 matches! A huge number to try and narrow down.

The profiles themselves are far more detailed than we'd imagined. You can't find out the donor's name, current location or an adult photo, but they have photos of them as a child, details about what they're like as a person, their family history and career information, a letter from them explaining why they wanted to be a donor (with a voice recording of them reading it) and results from intelligence and medical tests. There was even a part where the clinic gave their view on the donor and a comparison of their appearance to someone famous.

It felt really weird going into the first few profiles and scrutinising their life to see if we liked the sound of them. There were so many matches that we found ourselves starting to dismiss people quickly and over fairly trivial things, if they didn't sound like 'us' in personality or their letter didn't stand out enough. All completely surreal and not something we ever imagined doing.

We narrowed down the matches to a top ten first, then our three preferred, but there was always one profile that we connected with most. He was a Danish man and very similar to Rich in appearance, but the main draws were his questionnaire answers and personal letter. He liked the same things we did, he had three children and was described by the clinic as being 'a dedicated, hardworking family man'. In his letter, he told how a couple of his friends had trouble conceiving and how they'd used a donor. He saw the struggle they went through and wanted to help other couples become parents.

We loved the sound of his profile, but as advised by the clinic, we also kept the other two matches as back up, just in case our chosen donor hit their quota or the straws we needed became unavailable before we'd completed the process. With a sperm bank, each donor has 'straws' available that have different levels of motility. For our planned treatment, we'd been told we needed to have straws that had motility of 20 million and were also IUI-ready. Our chosen donor had enough at that level to cover three IUIs and an IVF cycle, and our clinic approved him to be a match with UK law.

Using a donor is a cost factor we hadn't considered at the start of our journey and we ended up spending £5000 on the straws, quota reservation and very specific international delivery. We're lucky to have incredibly supportive families and they generously gave us some money towards the unforeseen cost.

This was June 2019 and the delivery arrived at our clinic in time for us to have our first IUI attempt later that month. The odds were about 10-20% success rate, which didn't seem very high, but we had that naïve hope that it might work first time. It was an unmedicated cycle, so I just had a couple of scans from day 9 of my cycle to check the thickness of my womb lining and the follicle size to see when ovulation might be.

The process didn't seem that accurate to us – I had to monitor my own ovulation at home with Clearblue® tests and let the clinic know when I got the smiley face to say it was time. I'd had a scan on the Wednesday and they said ovulation wouldn't be for another few days based on my follicle size, but on the Thursday morning, I got a solid smiley face so I called them and they did the IUI procedure that afternoon. They didn't do another follicle scan to double check progress, and to me it didn't feel like the right time, even though the test said I was in the fertile window.

The procedure itself was straightforward: monitoring on an ultrasound screen, they used a thin catheter to place the sperm directly into my womb, and it only took five minutes. It was no more invasive than a smear test, and I didn't have many cramps afterwards. We sat in the clinic for about 15 minutes then went on our way, with instructions to take a pregnancy test in two weeks' time.

I instantly felt like it hadn't worked. I took some other ovulation tests that night and didn't get a strong positive until the next day, compared to the Clearblue® kit. I'd been hoping it would be a more accurate experience, although I guess it mimicked falling pregnant naturally, which doesn't have very high odds each month (knowing so much about the process now, I'm still amazed anyone conceives!). To us, it was a straw that cost £1250 though, and if it was unsuccessful, we decided not to proceed with the other two IUIs so we could use our remaining straws for future IVF treatment.

That two-week wait felt like forever. I was positive it hadn't worked, but every now and then I'd think, 'What if by some miracle it was the right time? What if the sperm lived long enough for the egg to release?'. I tried to symptom spot, but there wasn't anything. I took a test a couple of days before the date and we weren't surprised it was negative – even though there had always been that small hope deep down that we might be wrong, so it was still disappointing. I took another test on the date we'd been given, but by then we were just impatient to move forward with the next step.

Given how many years it took to get this stage, the treatment process actually moved really quickly for us once we had the donor chosen. I called the clinic to book in a follow-up appointment and they agreed to us moving straight onto IVF, which had a 30% success rate for my age.

After the IUI, we had a cycle break in July – although there are never really 'breaks' with infertility. It's always on your mind and I was still trying to prepare my body for the IVF cycle in August, with healthier eating, no alcohol and the right vitamins. We didn't really know much about the process, so did some research into what it would entail. I knew a couple of people who'd had IVF so we could ask them questions. And I found a lot of Instagram accounts to follow with ladies who had been through the process before or would be having transfers around the same time I would be (including several of the women in this book).

The online infertility community is amazing and I found so many people who knew what we were going through and would happily answer questions or offer their experiences. Our families and close friends knew we were starting IVF and were really supportive, but when you haven't been through it yourself, it's hard to fully understand the emotional and physical demand involved. Connecting with other women who knew what I was going through made the journey seem less daunting and like I had a strong support bubble. They don't refer to IVF women as 'warriors' for nothing.

Never having paid much attention to IVF before, I'd always assumed it was just a few hormone injections then they collected your eggs, made some embryos and you got pregnant first time (super naïve). In reality, it's far more complicated than that and there are absolutely no guarantees at any stage of the process.

As well as the hormone injections, there are also oestrogen pills and something I knew nothing about when I started (so they were a fun surprise!) progesterone pessaries. Three times a day for me... for 12 weeks if I became pregnant. There are different protocols for which drugs you take so it's a bit of a guessing game as to how your body will respond to stims. I was put on a fairly standard short protocol, which involved two injections most nights – one as a down regulation to suppress my own ovarian function and the other to stimulate follicle growth, to get as many eggs as possible. I was on Fyremadel® and Menopur®.

At the start, I was nervous about doing the injections myself. As Rich is a nurse, he did the first couple of days and showed me the best way to inject, until I was brave enough to try myself. I found it wasn't as difficult as I'd built up in my head. The second drug did sting though and I would always have a skin reaction with bright red bumps.

The injections have to be done at the same time every day, so the most interesting place I had to do them was at a wedding. I carried the two needles in my clutch bag in the day then injected them in the toilet during the reception, while Rich held my long dress out of the way – who said IVF wasn't glamorous!

I actually didn't feel too many side effects from my

cocktail of drugs, but I know several ladies who really suffered with mood swings, nausea and headaches. The progesterone also mimics symptoms of pregnancy, so it makes you second guess every little thing when you're waiting to find out if your transfer has been successful.

During the stims, I was having frequent scans to monitor how many follicles were growing. IVF is like a second job that you have to fit in around your day job. Luckily my design agency, Tickety Boo Creative (who designed this book cover), champion flexible working and were amazing at letting me work around my numerous appointments. Having an employer who I could be open with, and who offered me support, made me feel far more relaxed about the whole process and took away the stress of worrying about work colleagues covering for my absence or having to hide multiple appointments.

We also work from home full time (before the pandemic too), so that made things easier with getting to and from the clinic and being comfortable at home if I wasn't feeling great or recovering from procedures. I know a lot of people don't have that level of flexibility and support so I'm very grateful to the team I work with.

After a couple of weeks of monitoring, I had enough follicles measuring large enough to possibly contain mature eggs. In fact, I'd had a big surge in follicles that the doctors were concerned about. At my last scan, they counted 30 follicles and I was told there was a risk of Ovarian hyperstimulation syndrome (OHSS). Again, something I had never heard of. OHSS is an excessive response to the stims and around 33% of women undergoing IVF will have mild OHSS, but it can be very dangerous.

The clinic took a blood test so they could check my levels but told me that I was ready to take my trigger shot that evening (Tuesday), for an egg collection on the Thursday. The trigger injection signals your body to release the eggs and needs to be done exactly 36 hours before your egg retrieval operation.

I had to wait for the blood test results to confirm everything could go ahead as planned, but the results weren't what we'd hoped. My oestradiol levels were sky high: over 11,000 (far more than the 'ideal' range of 2,000-6,000 for IVF) and put me at huge risk for OHSS if our transfer was to go ahead, as the additional hormones if I got pregnant could make it even more severe.

I was given a different trigger drug to use so as not to make the situation any worse and they told us our fresh transfer would be cancelled and any embryos we had by day 5 would be frozen. We had to accept the situation for the sake of my health but it was so disappointing. We'd been excitedly counting down to the transfer and hoping that it might work. It felt like a huge blow to be told it couldn't go ahead and that we'd have to wait a couple of months for my body to recover before we could attempt a frozen embryo transfer. Plus, it would mean another cycle of drugs.

That night, we pulled the trigger for egg collection. The needle for that injection was enormous! We told our family and friends that unfortunately there wouldn't be a transfer, but we hoped we would get a few embryos to freeze.

On the morning of the egg collection, my stomach felt really swollen from all the follicles. I usually get a dull ache during ovulation from the side releasing the egg but this was a painful, constant ache across both ovaries.

We headed to the clinic and the retrieval went smoothly. I felt a little nervous going in, as I'd never had a procedure like that before and had no idea what to expect. They used mild sedation, rather than full anaesthetic, but I didn't remember anything about the process after they put the canula in my hand. It meant the recovery was quicker and compared to the constant aching pain I felt going into the collection, I was actually much more comfortable after.

The consultant came in a little while later and told us they'd retrieved 16 mature eggs. I knew that was a great number, but still felt a tiny bit disappointed as I'd had over 30 follicles (and through the flimsy curtain, we'd heard the couple next to us be told they had 19 eggs). They said they'd call us the next day to tell us how many fertilised overnight, then call on day 3 with progress, and again on day 5 to say how many embryos they'd be able to freeze.

We expected to lose eggs and embryos at each stage of the process so the number we'd be left with was a complete unknown. I'd heard of people losing half the amount at each stage, or not getting many that fertilised at the start, or not making it to day 5, so that made me nervous.

We headed home so I could relax, however the next morning, I got up and proceeded to break and dislocate my toe. I'd never broken anything before and I had to go to hospital to have an x-ray and my toe manipulated back into place. The break was clean but the pain of having my toe put back was far worse than the egg collection! I was sitting on the hospital bed, having my foot strapped, when the clinic rang. They told us that 13 of our eggs had fertilised and it was such a relief. We'd expected to lose more at the first stage so it felt like a good start. I hobbled home and took it easy for the rest of the day.

Waiting for the day 3 and day 5 calls was torture. My heart would start pounding every time my phone rang and I constantly panicked about how many embryos we'd get.

This was our only NHS-funded collection so we wanted to be left with enough for the three transfers – which would all now be FETs. I repeatedly looked up rough averages of how many embryos might survive the next step. On the days we were expecting a call, I would check my phone dozens of times in case I'd somehow missed the call, but at the same time, didn't want them to ring in case it was bad news.

When I saw the clinic's number on day 3, my hands started shaking. I tried to hear in the embryologist's voice whether it was good news. They told us that 11 embryos had made it to day 3! It was a really good number and more than we'd thought would make it that far, so it felt like a bit of the pressure was being lifted.

On day 5, they didn't call until late in the afternoon so naturally, I spent the day worrying we'd lost loads of the embryos. I kept telling myself if we ended up with 3-5 embryos to freeze that would be amazing. When they called, the embryologist told us that we had eight blastocysts (day 5 embryos) to freeze. I wanted to cry with relief. It was far more than we'd hoped for and more than enough for our transfers.

In the UK, they don't usually offer genetic testing on your embryos, unless it's something you ask and pay for specifically. PGS testing checks for abnormalities before transfer and can tell you the genders of the embryos, so we never knew which of ours were boys or girls, or how many were genetically 'normal'.

Months before treatment, we'd booked a Deep South tour of the US for September 2019. We'd debated booking anything around the time of treatment but we needed something to look forward to together and we hadn't had a break for a year. As our fresh transfer had been cancelled, we didn't have to worry about altering any activities if I'd been pregnant.

So much had been seemingly 'on hold' before the IVF cycle that it felt great to just go and enjoy ourselves and switch off for a bit before the FET. After nearly four years of TTC, it felt like a huge achievement to know we had eight frozen embabies waiting for us at home.

Our first FET was scheduled for my mid-October cycle. This cycle would be much easier on my body, with no stims for a collection, only oestrogen pills (to switch off my ovaries) and progesterone pessaries (to support the womb lining). There are some studies that show there's a slightly higher success rate with frozen transfers compared to fresh ones, as your body doesn't have full stims to recover from.

I took three pills and three pessaries each day and had a few scans to monitor my womb lining. Once it was thick enough to be a good environment for the embryo, they booked my transfer. It was another procedure I'd never experienced before so we didn't fully know what to expect.

On the day, they thawed our best quality embryo to transfer: a 5AB. The process is very quick, and quite similar to the IUI procedure. Using ultrasound, they find the best place to transfer, then the embryologist brings out a long, thin catheter containing the embryo. It's too small to see, so at the point of transfer a small air bubble is released, which looks like a little flash on screen, and means the embryo has been pushed through. The embryologist then takes the tube back into the lab to double check the embryo has definitely been transferred.

You need to have a full bladder for the procedure, to help the consultant find the right place for transfer. My bladder had felt full to me, but when they started scanning, they saw it was only three quarters full, so it took them a little while longer to get the angle right, and it did feel uncomfortable for a few minutes. It was weird being told to watch for the little white flash at the moment of transfer, knowing that was potentially our baby in there. Hoping that it would make a home for the next nine months.

This two-week wait was different to all the ones we'd experienced so far; this time we were PUPO (pregnant until proven otherwise). There was a great quality blastocyst in my uterus and a good chance of it sticking. Years of hard work had led up to this and the progesterone I was taking mimicked a few early pregnancy symptoms (nausea, tiredness, bloating), which meant we went back and forth each day on whether we thought it had worked or not. It really is an emotional rollercoaster. Some days I would think, 'Yep, it's definitely worked and I'm pregnant', other days I would be adamant it hadn't.

In hopes of helping the transfer take, we tried all the IVF remedies and superstitions we'd read about online. I ate pineapple each day for the bromelain, brazil nuts, McDonald's® fries (after transfer for the salt), I drank probiotics and Horlicks® for extra vitamins. I kept my feet constantly warm with thick socks and slippers. I didn't lift anything heavy or do any strenuous activity apart from some light walking. I even tried acupuncture, which I know a lot of people enjoy but it wasn't really my thing and I didn't find it relaxing at all.

I kept busy with work but it's hard to take your mind off what's happening inside your body. I'd thought I would be strong at the start and hold out until the date we'd been given to take a home pregnancy test (10 days after our transfer) but I couldn't do it. I had to know as soon as possible so I could stop the mental torture and potentially prepare myself for disappointment. Rich wanted to wait, but I caved and tested on day six, which was still early and might not show anything.

It was a BFN (big fat negative). The test had the same single line that I'd seen on dozens of other tests I'd taken over the years. I did the hopeful thing of taking the test into a different room and by the light of the window, squinting at the box to see if there was any hint of a second line. It was stark white.

There was a small chance the embryo had implanted late and the test could still change in a few days, but I knew deep down that it wouldn't. I told Rich it hadn't worked and could see the disappointment on his face. We'd both thought we might be lucky enough for it to work first time.

I took a couple more tests over the next few days but they were all negative and it was hard telling our family and friends that the transfer had failed. You don't normally have to update multiple people on your negative pregnancy tests and it felt extra deflating to disappoint the other people invested in our journey too. There was no reason for the transfer not to have taken, however in IVF nothing is a given. I knew that, but it still didn't stop me feeling guilty that my body had failed.

It wasn't only our best graded embryo we'd lost, it was months of effort, drugs, procedures, tears and hope. We'd imagined what that child might be like, whether they'd have been a boy or a girl, an entire future for them, then they were gone.

Calling the clinic was tough. They told us to stop taking our meds and wait for my period to arrive, then we would have an appointment to discuss next steps. While on the phone, I asked about the potential of the next cycle being in December. They usually like you to have a cycle break in between treatment, and from working out dates, I knew our next cycle would be mid-December, with a transfer around Boxing Day. The clinic closed over the Christmas period and they told us that unless our cycle started by the 3rd December (which it wouldn't) then our FET would be delayed until our mid-January cycle.

The thought of waiting another three months until the end of January for a transfer and getting through yet another Christmas and New Year of pregnancy announcements was too much. As an FET isn't as heavily medicated, we asked if there was any reason why we couldn't go back-to-back with cycles and have a transfer at the end of November instead. Our consultant was great and agreed that it was fine for us to do that, so they arranged to get new meds out to us quickly and booked the consent appointment for us to sign all the paperwork for the new transfer. It felt like a huge relief to know that we could try again straight away.

At our consent appointment a few days later, we asked if we could have two embryos transferred this time. We knew a few people who'd transferred two in the hope of increasing their chances of the transfer taking. They usually suggest two embryos if you've had multiple failed cycles, or if the embryos might have some quality issues, but again they agreed that we could. They explained the possibility of having multiple babies, as the pregnancy would become more high risk, and we still wanted to go ahead. They gave us only an 18% chance that both of them might implant, so it didn't seem too high.

The medication arrived in time and our second transfer came around fast: November 27th 2019. The day wasn't without some drama – we lost our second, best graded embryo during the thawing process. That was something I hadn't expected, months of effort lost in a second, never even making it to transfer. They thaw the embryos on the day, so they thawed another one in order to still transfer two. We were very lucky that we had more embryos, for some couples they might've only had one to transfer and it would've been cancelled. All the hope and emotion you invest in these cycles is completely out of your control.

We ended up transferring embryos that were graded 4AB and 4BA, one of which had thawed 100% and one only 90% but they thought it would catch up. Rich couldn't get out of work for the second transfer, so my mum actually came with me (pre-Covid). This time, I made sure my bladder was bursting before I went in and the procedure itself was much smoother. It took half the time of the first transfer and wasn't uncomfortable at all. We watched for the little flash of light and this time, the clinic gave me a photo of the exact moment so I could show Rich.

I still tried most of the remedies for the second transfer as I did in the first, so I don't know if any of those things actually work, but I do strongly believe that having my bladder extra full did help with the second transfer as my body was much more relaxed, rather than being tensed with the uncomfortable pain of them trying to get the right angle in the first one.

The two-week wait was torture again. For the first couple of days I was feeling positive – there were two little embryos so hopefully one of them would get comfy. Then the doubt started creeping in: what if it failed again? That would mean we'd lost four embryos in two months. Half of our precious embabies. If we had to do another FET, should we transfer two again, or just one, in the hope of not losing more than we had to? It's always hard to sleep during the long wait, with your brain constantly going back and forth, trying to guess what's happening inside your body.

I knew I would test early again; I hate not knowing. Our official test day was the Saturday, at 10dp5dt (10 days post 5-day transfer) but I took my first test on the

Wednesday… well, 1:15am on the Wednesday! It was close enough to 7dpt, when we should surely see something, and I couldn't cope with the uncertainty any longer. Rich had gone away for the night and if the test was positive, I really wanted to be able to surprise him when he came home. Something 'normal' that we hadn't been able to have at any point in our journey so far.

I'd planned to test at a more reasonable hour, with first-morning urine like recommended, but as I lay awake at 1am, I knew I had to test or I was never going to sleep. I hadn't really had any different symptoms to the same progesterone ones as the first transfer so I had no idea if it had worked.

I sat on the edge of the bath, with the test window facing away from me. My heart was pounding and it suddenly seemed too terrifying to find out what the result was. I took a deep breath and turned the test over. There were two, strong pink lines! The first positive test I had ever seen. There was no need to squint at the lines or question it, and after four long years I was hit by so many emotions – happiness, relief, fear. I started crying, and naturally, ended up not being able to sleep anyway because I was too excited.

I took another test as soon as I could – again, a strong double line. Then by 8am, I'd taken a third test – a digital one so I could see the word 'pregnant' for the first time. I then had to wait impatiently for Rich to get home later that day. I presented him with the positive tests, and it felt like we at last had a moment so many other couples get to just celebrate together.

We decided not to tell any of our family and friends that we were pregnant until after we'd doubled checked my HCG numbers with a blood test. Some UK clinics don't do beta tests, instead relying on your home pregnancy test results, but we wanted to have them for our own peace of mind, to make sure my numbers were ok and rising.

They knew our test day was the Saturday so we told people we hadn't tested early. It was extra hard hiding it from my parents though, after my mum had come to the transfer with me. To us, it felt like another little bit of normality we could have, to be in our own happy little bubble for a couple of days. IVF takes away any surprise. It's not the same as getting a positive test, waiting 12 weeks and then announcing your pregnancy (which I personally think is outdated – if something goes 'wrong' you shouldn't feel like you need to hide it. You should be able to grieve openly. A loss is a loss no matter what stage. Miscarriage happens to 1 in 4 women… 1 in 4, but it's not deemed acceptable to talk about it?!).

We went for a blood test at 8dpt and my HCG level came back at 311, which was really strong. I had a repeat beta the next day (Friday) at 9dpt, and the level was 521, so a big increase in 24 hours. For a viable pregnancy, they look for your number to double roughly every 48 hours. At this stage, we had no idea if one or both of the embryos had implanted, but the high rising level gave us a little glimmer of hope that it might be both of them.

Once we had the second number, we went to my parents' house to tell them. After so many years, it felt surreal to finally say out loud to other people that we were pregnant. There was a lot of excitement and tears, and we then told the rest of our family and close friends. The next morning, I took another digital test (just to test on official test day) and it upgraded to 'Pregnant 2-3 weeks', which was reassuring.

We excitedly called the clinic and were booked in for an early scan at exactly six weeks. With an IVF pregnancy, you have an early scan to check everything is progressing, then you 'graduate' to normal antenatal care by about 8-9 weeks. I couldn't wait to get to the scan and see the little baby/babies on the screen, to make the whole thing seem more real. I still didn't really have any symptoms, just a bit of trouble sleeping and feeling a little hungrier.

Unfortunately, the night before our 6-week scan, I had a huge bleed. It was bright red, fresh blood, and enough to fill the toilet. I was overcome with panic and we rushed to A&E, fearing the worst. I just kept thinking, how could we have gone through so much only to lose the baby this early, and the night before the first scan we'd been so excited for?

I was examined and the doctor told us it was a 'threatened miscarriage' but they couldn't give us any reassurance about which way things might go. There was no one who could scan me overnight so we had to wait until our fertility clinic scan the following day. Needless to say, it was the longest night ever and we got zero sleep. The bleeding continued, although not as much, and I had a few cramps but we were hoping the baby would hang on.

We got to the clinic the next day and I started crying as soon as the doctor took us into the room, sure it was going to be bad news. I closed my eyes as she started scanning, not wanting to see an empty screen. As soon as she moved the probe around though, she gave a little laugh and asked how many embryos we'd put in. I craned my neck to look at the screen and we were shocked to see two little gestational sacs. Twins!

There was a dark area directly underneath them, which was a pocket of blood, and explained why I was bleeding so much. Apparently, it can be more common with a multiple pregnancy.

The babies were slightly too small for heartbeats at that stage (one had the tiniest little flicker) and were measuring 5w6d (5 weeks 6 days) and 6w1d, so they booked us in for another scan at 7w4d so we could check on progress. We left the room in a bit of a daze, having gone from tears of despair to tears of joy in the space of a few minutes.

It was the best feeling to be able to tell our family and friends that not only were we still pregnant, we were expecting twins. That was five days before Christmas, so we spent the festive period celebrating our amazing news and excitedly making plans for the future.

The bleeding continued on and off, which worried me every time I went to the toilet, and I still didn't have many pregnancy symptoms. I was lucky enough not to get any morning sickness, but to me it seemed like a really bad thing, as I would worry it was a sign that things weren't ok.

The day before New Year's Eve we had our second scan, and it was the only one I went in to feeling excited. But as soon as the scan started, we could tell something was wrong. One of the babies dwarfed the other in size and there was only one heartbeat. They told us that sadly one of the babies had stopped growing at 6 weeks. They said it was called vanishing twin syndrome and unfortunately common in multiple pregnancies.

It was devastating to hear and felt like a very strange mix of emotions to feel grief for losing one baby, while still being happy to be pregnant with another. We were so grateful to have one baby growing well, but once we'd known there were two, we'd wanted both of them. We'd been dreaming of how our life would look with twins. It was gut wrenching to have to tell our close friends and family bad news once more: that one of the babies hadn't made it. We didn't even know if that baby was a boy or girl.

They booked us in for one last scan at 8w4d to

graduate the fertility clinic. I was absolutely petrified that this time we'd be told the other baby hadn't made it either. That we would have to cope with two losses and somehow find the strength to move forward with another FET in the future. It was the start of the 'scanxiety' that plagued me through the rest of the pregnancy, stemming from the trauma of the first two scans. I would count down to each scan, and then not be able to sleep for days before. After so many years of hearing negative outcomes from infertility, we would just expect the worst at every step.

Rich couldn't get out of work for the third scan, so my dad actually came with me. The staff were a little surprised – I don't think many people bring their dad with them to the fertility clinic! But I'm very close to my parents and they're so supportive. In a way, it was nice they got to be involved in the journey they were so invested in.

I felt terrified when the doctor started scanning, steeling myself to hear more bad news. She was quiet for a minute as she moved the probe around and I could see two babies on the screen that seemed to be the same size. At first, I was confused and thought, 'Oh god, the other one has stopped growing too'. But then we realised there were two strong heartbeats! Two moving babies! The doctors were so surprised that three of them came to see, including the one who'd scanned us the week before. The babies were now both measuring right on track, with the smaller one having grown at twice the speed. They were so happy for us and said it was rare to have such a late developing baby. We graduated from the clinic and I left the fertility department for the last time.

I phoned Rich the second I left the clinic, so he immediately panicked that something was wrong. I was a mess and all I could get out was: 'The baby is back!'. He couldn't believe it! The rollercoaster of emotions had continued from IVF into the pregnancy and we felt exhausted. Those three weeks had been more draining than the three treatment cycles before. Once again, we had to update our close friends and family, but this time with the good news that we were having twins again.

We were more cautious in celebrating though, worried about how quickly things had changed before. I was desperate to get to the 12-week scan to make sure they were both still there. Now we were under normal antenatal care, I had my midwife booking in appointment at 9 weeks. They were really nice and after hearing about our infertility journey and the vanishing/not vanishing twin they booked me in for a scan at the EPAU, just to check both babies were still doing ok. I was still having some bleeding, which continued until I was about 17 weeks pregnant, with several large bleeds again just to make things that bit more tense.

Thankfully both babies were growing well at nearly 10 weeks, then it was time for the first big scan at 12 weeks. It was back up at our clinic again, but this time on the maternity floor instead of the fertility one. We'd spent years there dreaming of one day getting into the lift and being able to go up to the second floor, so it felt like a huge moment to finally press the '2' button. Again, I was scared before the scan and held my breath until they'd checked that both babies had heartbeats. They were doing well and it was amazing to see them moving about on the screen.

The sonographer turned to us about halfway through and asked if we were going to find out the sex of the babies. We'd always wanted to find out so we said yes, thinking we'd be able to see at the 20-week scan. She then pointed to the screen and said, 'Well, he's showing us' and laughed. We were so surprised they could see that early but it was pretty clear the baby was a boy! They thought the other baby was 70% a girl but would need to wait to confirm (they were right on both counts).

The pregnancy itself progressed well but waiting until the 20-week scan to see the babies again felt like such a long time, even though we'd become accustomed to waiting through our infertility journey. The bleeding still made me panic every time I went to the toilet, so we booked to have a private scan at 18 weeks for some reassurance, and to confirm if the genders had been correct. I'm so glad we booked that scan, because only two days after it, the UK went into lockdown due to the COVID-19 pandemic. It meant that was the last scan Rich could attend with me for the rest of my pregnancy, and the last time things felt 'normal'.

The infection numbers had been getting increasingly worse, so we knew something big was about to happen, but not how much it would impact our lives. As Rich is an NHS nurse, he was redeployed from cardiology to run a respiratory HDU, treating very ill Covid patients. For the safety of the babies and myself, we had to distance from each other for months while he was so exposed. He worked extra-long shifts and we barely saw each other. We slept in different rooms, and he was extra careful with full PPE and washing and changing as soon as he got home, but we still didn't have any contact just in case.

I worked from home, locked-down like everyone else, and grew our two babies. After so many years of trying, it was not the pregnancy we'd always dreamed of. I couldn't see anyone apart from video calls, no one saw my bump growing, and there was suddenly a huge gap in my maternity care.

I went to the 20-week scan alone, then I didn't have another appointment until I was 28 weeks and had my first twins' clinic. Instead of midwife appointments, I had a couple of brief phone calls where they asked if everything was ok and I said, 'I think so', not sure I would have any idea if it wasn't. Even though it was my first pregnancy and high risk with twins, I didn't have my blood, urine or blood pressure checked for weeks. It felt as if I'd been robbed of standard pregnancy care and it added extra stress with worrying about the babies.

The rollercoaster first nine weeks, and the impact of so many years of infertility, meant I didn't enjoy pregnancy as much as I'd always thought I would. We were so grateful to be pregnant, but there was a constant, underlying feeling of anxiety, knowing everything it had taken for us to finally conceive. I constantly set milestones in my head of dates I wanted to reach and then I could 'relax'. First it was 12 weeks, then 20 weeks, then 24 weeks for viability, then 28 weeks to give the babies more chance and so on. Rich would wait for me to get to the specified week and then set the next milestone.

Thankfully, things with the pandemic eased a little about four weeks before the twins made an early appearance, and we were able to have a couple of socially distanced, outdoor baby showers with some family and friends. It felt amazing to finally be able to have people see my 30-week bump and feel like we could celebrate.

Physically, my pregnancy went well. There wasn't too much tiredness, I could still walk the dog every day and I worked up until I was 33w5d. As I approached 34 weeks, the complications began: the rib pain became unbearable, my blood pressure sky rocketed and I had one severely swollen leg, which they thought might be a blood clot.

I went into hospital for monitoring at 34w3d and my waters broke as soon as I got to the maternity ward. I immediately started worrying whether the babies would need special care if they were born that prematurely.

They tried to hold off labour with a hormone patch and I had a steroid injection to strengthen the babies' lungs.

As with most of our journey, the birth didn't go how we'd hoped. I was examined the following night, after some bleeding, and there was chaos. They said I was 9cm dilated and had to get to delivery immediately as they could feel twin 1's head coming. People started throwing my belongings onto the bed and I was wheeled down the corridor while I frantically called Rich to tell him to get to the hospital as fast as he could. I just kept thinking, 'This can't be right, I haven't even had a contraction, how can the babies be coming?'.

When someone more senior examined me in delivery, it turned out I was only 4-5cm dilated, but our little boy's head was so small it had seemed like more. We decided to try for a natural birth, but after 15 hours and a hormone IV, I remained stuck at 8cm so we needed an emergency c-section.

In an amazing twist of fate, our doctor from the fertility clinic now worked as an obstetrician at our local hospital, and he was on shift that afternoon. So, the man who helped to create our babies got to deliver them too, which was just incredible.

The c-section itself went well and the babies were born at 16:48 and 16:50. Unfortunately, after the delivery I haemorrhaged and ended up losing 2.5L of blood and needed six transfusions. I was reopened under general anaesthetic and had my womb stitched around to compress it back down, with a temporary drain out through my stomach. Needless to say, it was a far more terrifying and traumatic experience than we'd expected.

Four hours later, I finally got to hold our babies. Our little boy, Christopher, weighed 4lb 10oz, and our girl, Amara, was 5lb 12oz. We'd chosen the names fairly early in the pregnancy – as soon as we'd been told one baby was a boy, Rich wanted to call him Christopher after our lovely friend Chris.

Amazingly, they didn't need any special care and could stay with me on the ward. With Covid restrictions, Rich could only come and visit us for four hours in the afternoons, otherwise I was alone with the babies until we were finally all allowed home after a week.

Due to the pandemic, my maternity leave also hasn't been what I'd always dreamed during so many years of TTC. We've spent the seven months since the babies were born in various forms of lockdown. There have been no baby clubs, no swimming classes, no playdates with my friends and family. Rich had to go back to treating Covid patients again during the rise after Christmas, which meant more long hours away from us.

I do worry that it'll affect the babies. They don't really know anyone else and cry when they see other people or go to other places. I'm hoping they'll adapt well once they start being allowed to do more when the restrictions lift.

Reflecting on our journey now, we've been through so much over the last five years and I'm so unbelievably grateful that we have our beautiful babies. I love watching their little personalities shine through and seeing them grow and develop. They're doing so well and we couldn't love them more. One day, we'll tell them about how they came into the world and talk to them openly about donor conception, and hopefully they'll be able to read this book when they understand more. This journey is only a small part of who they are and who they will be, but we hope they'll be proud of it, and know how much they were wanted.

We will always be infertile though; having children doesn't change that fact. There will never be a surprise pregnancy in our lives. If we do decide we want another child in the future (which doesn't seem likely at the moment), then we would need to have another FET. We have four embryos still frozen at the clinic, which I do think about sometimes. We don't know how long we'll keep them frozen for, whether we'll ever have another transfer, or whether it would even work if we did.

This journey has taken so much from us emotionally and physically, and I'm so glad that Rich and I have a strong relationship and we've supported each other throughout (and had incredible support from our family and friends). I know that isn't always the case, so we're very lucky in that respect. We were so naïve at the start though and had no idea what infertility could entail. That was one of the reasons I wanted to reach out to the ladies in this book to share their stories, to hopefully raise more awareness and support other women and couples in this community, while raising money for related charities too. No one's journey or outcome is the same, but the infertility community is so supportive and we hope this will help other people know that they aren't alone.

Rich

Often when researching infertility and the journey through IVF, it's the testimonials of the mother at the top of the searches. Generally, I think that the mother's journey is talked about more because we (men) don't want to talk about it openly. After all, there's nothing more emasculating than 'firing blanks' and not being able to have children of your own – I know I don't like talking about it!

But, having been through the journey of tests, surgery and disappointments, the ups and downs of IVF, the heartbreak of failure and loss, and the feeling of pure elation at the end of it all (which is actually just the beginning), I've realised how much better I'd have coped if I had talked about it as it was happening.

Looking back on all of it, I don't ever regret agreeing to all the tests and starting the IVF process but f**k me was it exhausting! Made all the more tiring by having that thought in the back, and often the front of my mind: 'These kids aren't going to be biologically mine'. I was obsessed with the idea that because we had to use a donor, the baby/babies wouldn't have any of me in them and I therefore wouldn't bond with them. Looking at my twin son and daughter now that whole idea seems ridiculous, I'm their dad, and they know it! Christopher somehow even looks just like me.

There's a lot in the media at the moment about men's mental health and it's always been something we've pretty much ignored. Not because we think we're fine, but because we know we're not and have decided that this is as good as it gets. But maybe talking about it will help? Not to a counsellor or a professional, but to those who are going through the same shit we are. I don't pretend to be an expert on male coping mechanisms through IVF, but if this helps just one person then it's worth it. So, keep your peckers up!

Chosen charity

Our charity is Fertility Network UK:
fertilitynetworkuk.org

They provide information, advice, support and understanding for those dealing with infertility. They're also affiliated with the HIMfertility campaign to help raise awareness of male factor infertility and offer support to men.

Katy and Tom

After five and a half years of TTC, four treatment cycles and three losses, they are finally expecting their rainbow baby boy in May 2021. They talk about their experiences with IVF, unexplained infertility, baby loss/miscarriage, failed cycles and pregnancy after IVF and loss.

Katy

My name is Katy, I am 29 and a healthcare assistant. I live in Devon, England with my husband, Tom, who's 31 and has recently left the military to pursue a career in accounting. I also live with my beautiful dog, Stan, who is 14 years young – I've had him since I was 15, so he is my baby.

I share my story in the hope that it can help others and raise awareness. Like many, we have been on this long journey for five and a half years. We started trying to conceive in 2015. We fell pregnant naturally for the first time and we were over the moon that it happened so quickly after me coming off the contraceptive pill. I wouldn't say we were actively trying – we'd been engaged for 18 months (no wedding planned yet) and we had the thought process of 'if it happens, it happens', like a lot of couples. When we found out I was pregnant, we brought our wedding forward to April and everything seemed to be going smoothly.

We went to our 12-week scan (which was two weeks before our wedding), and I remember seeing our baby on the screen so clearly and thinking, 'This baby isn't the size of a 12-week pregnancy', it was more like the size of an 8-week pregnancy. I knew this because a close friend of mine at the time had an early scan and they were a similar size. When the sonographer called someone else into the room, I knew something was wrong. We were then told that our sweet baby had no heartbeat. I'd experienced a missed miscarriage.

We both completely broke down. It felt like our lives were shattered and all the plans we'd made, all the dreams, were just gone in a flash. That was the day that changed us forever. I don't think we've been the same ever since but it has made us stronger over time. I opted for a D&C; I just wanted it to be over with. After having no signs of a miscarriage beforehand, I didn't want to wait and see if nature would take its course. However, looking back, I wish I hadn't jumped to that decision so quickly, as I always blame those operations as a reason why we couldn't conceive in the future.

We got married two weeks later. I went into a numb zone, I had the wedding to think about, whereas Tom was able to grieve straight away. It always takes me a few months and then it finally hits me hard. We had the best intimate wedding with a small number of friends and family. It was such a lovely day, but every time I look at pictures, it just reminds me of how broken we were at that time in our lives. We have always said we would have a vow renewal at 10 years, hopefully with our children beside us.

After a difficult year struggling with what had happened and trying to move on from it all, I was desperately trying to get pregnant again. Exactly a year after our loss, I fell pregnant. We were so happy and excited, thinking 'this is our time' and surely it couldn't happen again. However, at around six weeks pregnant I had spotting, which is very common but deep down I knew something wasn't right. I went to the EPU and they did a scan, which showed the gestational sac but no yolk sac or fetal pole. I was just past six weeks so I knew there should've been something but I was told it was too early and to come back a week later. We came back a week later and still nothing to be seen; again, I was told it could still be early.

Then one morning, I had just woken up at home and I got a phone call from a doctor saying I needed to come to the hospital straight away. He sounded panicked and then said, 'We think you're having an ectopic pregnancy'. Tom was away with the military at the time and it was very difficult to get hold of him to come home. I went in to hospital on my own and Tom would join me later. When I got to the hospital, they all seemed to be in a bit of a panic – rushing me through, getting a canula put in my arm and making sure I hadn't eaten. They showed me to a bed and the doctor arrived with a consent form, saying they would like to do a laparoscopy. They thought I was having an ectopic pregnancy because my blood HCG levels weren't coming down. I signed the consent forms, which meant I was signing away my fallopian tubes if they did find anything. It was all a bit surreal because my mum had an ectopic pregnancy before me, and that is the reason she went on to have me through IVF.

I waited all day for the procedure and during that time, the nurses and doctors kept asking me if I was in pain (which I wasn't at all) and whether I had been bleeding (which I hadn't been). I knew I wasn't having an ectopic pregnancy and to this day, I am convinced they got me mixed up with someone else.

Tom eventually arrived and I went into theatre that evening. They opened me under general anaesthetic and the procedure only lasted about 5-10 minutes. I woke up and I remember the nurse (who I knew from working in that hospital) saying, 'Good news, it isn't ectopic'. After my time in recovery, they sent me home, explaining that it wasn't an ectopic pregnancy and there was a clear gestational sac in my uterus, so to come back in a week's time – at this point I was about 7-8 weeks pregnant.

My follow up with the specialist nurse who'd seen me previously was a week later and she was furious. She was so angry they'd operated on me when she'd specifically said in her notes that there was no sign of an ectopic pregnancy – she could see the tubes were clear from an ultrasound. She said they'd given me unnecessary surgery, which of course, made us angry too. She continued to scan me and we still had the same results – there was a sac with no fetal pole or yolk sac. This went on for many weeks. I kept going back each week and getting the same result but the guidelines at our hospital stated that until I was 12 weeks with no sign of a fetal pole, then they couldn't say whether it was a viable pregnancy or not.

At 12 weeks, they decided it wasn't going to be viable. I was relieved, as I was so fed up and I'd known the pregnancy wasn't viable from day one. Finally, someone made the decision and diagnosed me with a blighted ovum (where a sac and placenta grow but a baby doesn't). After my body didn't reject or realise there was an issue again, and after so long, I decided to have another D&C. I was exasperated and I wanted to get back to normal as soon as possible.

After two more difficult years of trying to conceive naturally again, we had no success. It was such a tough couple of years. I look back now and I can definitely say I was depressed. I was not in a good way at all. I couldn't speak to anyone about it, nor did I know anyone else who had experienced pregnancy loss or anyone struggling to conceive no one who was open about it anyway.

After seeking help from my GP, we had the initial fertility tests, such as checking my hormone levels at different times of the month to make sure I was ovulating and everything came back within normal range. We were then referred to the fertility clinic. We had a few more tests – a HyCoSy for me (Hysterosalpingo contrast sonography, which is an investigation of the fallopian tubes and cavity of the uterus) and a semen analysis for Tom – which also came back normal. Our fertility doctor diagnosed us with unexplained infertility, which affects approximately 1 in 5 couples who are trying to conceive.

A diagnosis of unexplained infertility was really frustrating – we would've liked a reason as to why getting pregnant naturally wasn't happening for us, but at the same time, we were grateful there wasn't anything serious and nothing stopping us from getting pregnant. We had very mixed emotions. With our diagnosis, we still tried to conceive naturally. We still did a pregnancy test every single month, only to feel the heartbreak each time it was negative. We were no closer to being pregnant again.

Our fertility consultant referred us for IVF. We came under the NHS England funding for IVF as Tom was in the military at the time, which we were very grateful for. It meant we could have three rounds of IVF and any frozen transfers in between, which really is amazing. We started our IVF journey at the end of 2018. At the same time, I found the amazing TTC community online, which has helped me so much.

I was surprised to find the medication side effects were not as bad as I thought. I started my cycle with down regulation and one of the medications, Norethisterone, really did not suit me though. I had all the symptoms of menopause from that drug but I powered through, carrying on as normal with everyday life, which was difficult but you have to. We both had a 'go with the flow' attitude at the beginning of IVF, and I remember it being exciting at first. My parents had conceived me through IVF all those years ago and it had worked first time for them, so we were convinced it would work first time for us.

During stimulation, I knew I had quite a lot of follicles on one side as I could feel it. It was such a strange feeling but we got the go ahead to have retrieval a few days later. I was awake for the retrieval. I had a Voltarol® pessary and some pain relief through a cannula, but I knew exactly what was going on. I lay on the bed and the embryologist performing the retrieval kept counting each egg they managed to retrieve – it was exciting. I was then wheeled back to the recovery area and waited. We didn't know how many mature eggs we had got at this point. I heard the embryologist come in, about to chat to us, but then we were told to join him in another room. I always fear the worst when any medical person tells you they want to chat in a room, so we began to get nervous.

We sat in the room and the embryologist explained that Tom's sperm sample from that day wasn't as good as his previous samples. My heart sank – I hadn't thought that would be a problem, all I'd been thinking about were my eggs and numbers. He explained that the sperm morphology results weren't what they'd hoped but he wasn't overly concerned, which was good news. They advised us to have a 'split cycle'. This meant half of our eggs would be fertilised the conventional way and the other half would be fertilised using ICSI (something else I didn't know anything about), but we were happy to go with their advice.

The embryologist told us he'd retrieved 17 eggs, which was great, but again, I hadn't done any research as to what happened next – we were very naïve and didn't have a clue. I sometimes wish it was all explained more to us but at the same time, I look back and think I know too much now that I would've stressed about numbers. Out of our 17 eggs, eight were fertilised with ICSI (of which five fertilised) and eight using conventional IVF (of which three fertilised) and we had one egg not maturing at all. I remember feeling awful at the time, as it feels like you've lost so many eggs after going through so much to get them. Now I know more about IVF, we were very lucky to get the amount of eggs we did.

They monitored our eggs daily and by day 5, we had five top quality blastocysts, with the possibility of two more catching up. We were very happy as this meant we would have a few chances at IVF. It also meant we could have a fresh transfer on day 5 so, on 21st January 2019, we transferred one 5AA ICSI embryo, while the other four embryos were frozen.

Transfer was so surreal. On this particular occasion, I didn't see the embryo flash on the screen when it went in but I remember feeling that 'I've got to protect this embaby', it was a nice cosy feeling. I had the usual McDonald's® fries, which to me was the perfect excuse. When I went for a wee afterwards, I literally thought the embryo would fall out! Even walking to the car or driving over bumps in the road, I thought it would move the embryo into the wrong place. The things that run through your head – even when I coughed, I thought it would damage the embryo – but rest assured, none of these things can harm your embryo. The next day, we got the call that one of the two remaining embryos was able to be frozen, which was amazing and we then had five frosties (frozen embryos).

I didn't do much after transfer. Thankfully, I was able to have the two-week wait off work so I just relaxed and ate healthily. Unfortunately, five days after transfer, I started bleeding. I knew this wasn't good news but the clinic still told me to take the test on official test day and it was a negative. It was devastating. You feel like you've mentally and physically put yourself through so much, only for it to end five days later – what was the point? It felt like a waste and we were absolutely gutted. We began to feel like it would never happen for us.

A few months passed, and at our WTF appointment ('What the f**k' follow-up appointment, lovingly named by the TTC community) we discussed whether there was anything to change with the FET protocol. By this point, I'd followed many journeys on social media and had talked to many other warriors going through IVF. I was convinced the first transfer hadn't worked because the Cyclogest® pessaries were not enough for me. I also felt they weren't absorbing properly and this was the reason my previous cycle ended only five days after transfer. The consultant agreed that we could try Lubion® progesterone injections instead.

We started our first FET in April 2019, again with a down regulation protocol using Norethisterone tablets (which I hated) and Buserelin injections. We'd had our down regulation scan booked in to check my lining was thin enough and my ovaries had essentially been shut down, but I hadn't had a bleed by the time the scan arrived. Typical – when you don't want your period to arrive, it arrives, and when you really want it to, it doesn't! Thankfully, it arrived a few days later and I was able to start the next part of the cycle.

I started oestrogen tablets to thicken up my lining ready for transfer. I had my first lining scan 10 days later but unfortunately, my lining was only 6.2mm and they wanted it to be at least 7mm. It meant my transfer week wasn't going ahead as planned. There are so many setbacks in the process, which is frustrating and I built myself up for things to go as planned, only for it to change. Four days later, they checked my lining again and it was still only 6.9mm, but not far off what they wanted, so they decided to add oestrogen patches to go alongside the tablets. Thankfully, another four days later my lining was a great 8.3mm, so they scheduled transfer for five days' time. I started progesterone injections that evening, which were sore at first but I got used to them.

Transfer went as planned, on the 29th May 2019 with an ICSI embryo. We did all the same routine after transfer and the two-week wait began. This time, I didn't bleed at five days, which was a positive, however on official test day it was a BFN (Big fat negative). We were absolutely devastated again. It is just so exhausting, all the emotions, all the hope, only to be left with nothing afterwards. We were told to wait a couple of days to test again, which was torture. I just wanted it to end. I knew it was over; it was still a negative so we stopped all medication and I had a bleed soon after.

We had our WTF appointment in July 2019 and it's so frustrating when they can't tell you why it's failed. I even got told that one in three transfers work, so we were thinking next time would be third time lucky. I suggested having an endometrial scratch with the next transfer – which is a procedure to 'scratch' the lining of the womb in the hope of triggering your body to repair the site, releasing chemicals and hormones that make the womb lining more receptive to an embryo implanting. At this point, I wanted to try everything and thankfully the consultant agreed. We were lucky that this transfer would be with the NHS funding still. We also decided that I would start the oestrogen patches straightaway, instead of having the delay in my lining thickening, and continue with Lubion®, as it had helped me not have an early bleed.

We started our second FET in September 2019. I had the same issue with not having a bleed in time for my down regulation scan but my lining did get thick enough in time, by using the patches straightaway. Our transfer was due to go ahead on 10th October and I remember waiting for that dreaded phone call on the morning of transfer, to see if our embryo had thawed successfully. That's such a fear and this time, they did actually say that our first conventional IVF embryo hadn't thawed as well as they had hoped, but it was still a good embryo. They gave us the option to thaw another embryo (which I thought was great if they could transfer two), but being under the criteria of NHS England funding in our area, they said that if the other embryo was better quality they could still only transfer one. This seemed like a waste to us and we were upset, so we decided not to thaw out another embryo and go ahead with the transfer.

This time, we saw the flash of the embryo going in and it was such a lovely experience. We can honestly say it felt different – we had a completely different team and it felt more relaxed. The two-week wait was here again. The only difference was I'd had my fries the night before because I'd just wanted to get home after transfer and relax. After two failed transfers, we'd become impatient so we tested early. To be honest, I did feel a little different so six days after transfer, we tested and it was a positive!! We had so many mixed emotions. We hadn't seen a positive test for over four years.

We told our family it had worked and Tom would

have his 30th birthday celebrations that week too. We were very cautious, as we'd miscarried twice previously, so we took a test every day. It was ok for a couple of days but then the tests started to get lighter, which wasn't a good sign. On OTD (official test day), it was still positive so we had hope. It wasn't as strong as it had been though and three days after OTD, it was negative – unfortunately, we were having a chemical pregnancy. What made it worse was by the time the doctor did a blood test, my HCG levels were so low he claimed it hadn't worked in the first place. That was devastating – such hope and excitement only for it to disappear 10 days later. I think at this point we were ready to give up. I couldn't put myself through it again. My mum had just been diagnosed with pancreatic cancer and I really wanted her to be around to find out if it was successful, or even hoped she would be here to see her grandchild. That's what kept me positive and determined to keep going.

We enjoyed Tom's 30th celebrations and also festivities over Christmas. We had our WTF appointment in December 2019, by this point we were one year in to IVF with no success. We agreed to have one more investigation so I had a hysteroscopy. I was convinced that after having two D&Cs they'd maybe damaged something. I was desperate for them to find something to explain why we weren't getting pregnant naturally or through IVF. I had the procedure and there was nothing to be found, everything looked normal. Which of course, was great news, but also frustrating.

With everything looking normal (and the agreement not to start with Norethisterone, as I thought it was delaying my bleed during down regulation), we started treatment for our third FET in February 2020. We started with another endometrial scratch, as we'd got a bit further in our cycle last time, so we agreed to give it another go.

Three weeks into treatment (and taking the Buserelin injections), and on the day of my down regulation scan, I got a phone call to tell me that due to the pandemic, all cycles were cancelled. I was absolutely devastated. You wait so long in between treatments and leading up to starting treatment, all that preparation to be told it's no longer going ahead. It was such a scary time as I work in the hospital myself, so I knew it was for the best, but I felt lost again, not really knowing when we could start treatment. I look back now and I'm glad my cycle got cancelled, as I did actually get Covid myself in March 2020 and that would've been around the time of transfer.

After months of waiting, and so many infertility community members advocating for fertility treatments to be restarted, including me sharing my story on the news (which was a little surreal), the secretary of state for health announced that on the 11th May 2020, all clinics could apply to reopen. This was fantastic news for many men and women across the country.

Our clinic took a little longer but they were able to open and we had a telephone consultation mid-June 2020. We were told we could restart our third FET on our next cycle. We were over the moon with this news, finally we were able to look forward again. By the time we transferred our next embryo, it had been 11 months since our last transfer – which was a long break but it did me the world of good. Aftcr thc news that everything got cancelled, I started a couch to 5K programme and I developed a love for running. It helped me so much mentally and physically. I also started a Fad Free For Life diet, which completely changed my mindset on what I was eating.

We had another endometrial scratch and started the medication again in July 2020, and this time, I had a bleed on time (thanks to stopping the Norethisterone tablets). It felt like such a long protocol – I was actually taking Buserelin injections for five weeks and I could really feel it. My lining was perfect for transfer on the exact date they wanted it to be and then, instead of getting the news that planned transfer week would go ahead, the clinic decided to put it back a week because there was a staff shortage due to Covid. I was furious and so upset – for once everything had been going to plan. It meant I had to be on those injections for another week and it also meant I had to take time off sick at work because I'd been told to self-isolate two weeks prior to transfer. I soon got over it though and calmed myself down in preparation for our transfer.

In the week leading up to transfer, we were given an option from the embryologist. We had one day 5 borderline blastocyst (ICSI), one day 5 optimal blastocyst (ICSI) and one day 6 hatching blastocyst (conventional IVF). She gave us the option of which one we would like to transfer, or they would make the decision for us. We ended up deciding to go with the day 6 embryo, because it was an IVF embryo and our previous transfer that resulted in the positive test had been an IVF embryo. We also quite liked the idea of it already hatching and knowing it powered on that extra day after egg collection. Usually an embryologist wouldn't choose a day 6 over a day 5, but we got to decide and that's exactly what we chose.

Transfer went ahead on 2nd September. It all went smoothly and I saw the flash of the embryo going in again. Unfortunately, due to Covid restrictions, Tom wasn't able to be in the room with me, which was upsetting but we understood.

We had the usual fries the night before again and I relaxed the day of transfer, but this time I was more active. I made sure I went out for a walk every day during the two-week wait – I'd read something about it being great to get the blood flowing. We carried on as normal, going out for a couple of meals which was nice. After last time, I'd been determined not to take a test early but then I was chatting to another lady who'd had a transfer the day before me and she got a positive on day 4! I had tests in the house (which I know I shouldn't as it's too tempting) so I took a test at 4dp6dt too. It was positive! We couldn't believe it had worked again. Symptom-wise, throughout the TWW I'd had a mild headache, my dreams were a bit more vivid and I'd had mild cramps, slight nausea and sore boobs, although this could have been from the progesterone mimicking symptoms.

Tom wouldn't believe it until official test day, but I was taking pregnancy tests daily and the line was getting darker this time, not lighter like before. On OTD it was still a very strong positive and we were ecstatic but also anxious. Could this actually be our time? Or would it end in the first trimester, like all the other times?

Just before six weeks pregnant, I had some brownish spotting and the fear set in again – it had always been bad news for us after seeing spotting. I called the clinic and although they said it was very common, I insisted on having blood tests and an early scan. It was still early for a scan but they did bloods at my local hospital and my HCG had nearly doubled like it should. Still not convinced, as that's what pregnancy after loss makes you feel like, we waited for our scan. It was terrifying. We went in to the ultrasound room and thankfully Tom was able to be there with me. On the screen, there it was

– the tiniest little dot with a beating heart and everything where it should be. Tom squeezed my arm and I burst into tears. After five years, this was the first time we had seen a heartbeat. It was like it was a dream.

Pregnancy after loss is another journey in itself, even pregnancy after years of infertility is the same. We really didn't believe it was happening. In the early days, I wouldn't allow myself to be happy or get excited. I kept pushing the goalpost, saying when we get to such and such week I could relax, but the truth is, I don't think you ever do until they're here. Even then, someone told me you won't relax again once you become a mum.

We must have had over 10 scans! Family joked, saying that he/she is the most photographed baby before they're even born. Even the private clinic joked with us, saying we were paying for their Christmas do, but to us it was more than just seeing him/her, it was the reassurance that everything was looking fine and healthy. That's all that mattered. Our nickname for baby is 'Hatchy Pants', because it was the embryo that was already hatching and the one we chose.

We had a 16-week private scan to find out the gender of our baby but we didn't find out then, we wanted Tom's mum to tell us on Christmas Day with a gender reveal. We sent the gender in the post without looking (trust me, that took some will power) but it was all worth it when we found out the news on Christmas Day. We pulled a canon outside so everyone could join and I had my mum on FaceTime. It was such a special moment and a Christmas I will never forget.

We're having a boy! It felt so much more real to us when we knew what we were having – like he's a little person. We were able to start buying things for him and start his nursery, and it was all starting to feel more exciting. I started feeling him kick, which was all the reassurance I needed. It is finally happening for us and every single night we actually say to each other: 'We are having a baby'. I honestly don't think we'll believe it until he's here.

As I mentioned, my mum was diagnosed with stage 4 pancreatic cancer back in 2018. She had been there through everything with me, and after going through IVF herself, she knew exactly how I was feeling. She used to say, 'Right, now let's move on. Keep smiling and try again'. Which we did. I was determined to make sure she was here to be able to see her grandchild. She fought so hard and was an absolute warrior but unfortunately, when I was 28 weeks pregnant, she sadly passed away.

I'm thankful that she was able to see all of his scans and even feel him kick. She also wrote in his baby shower book, which means the world to me, and having her just know that we are going to be ok. As I write this, it has only been a few weeks since her passing, so I don't know what navigating through birth or motherhood will be like without my mum, but I do know she will be looking down on us and protecting us.

Our baby boy is due in May 2021. We do have a name chosen, as I wanted my mum to know it too. We have nearly finished his nursery and are slowly preparing to become the best parents we can be. We are looking forward to his arrival and we're just so grateful we have finally been given this chance. Our future is welcoming our baby boy in May and navigating our way through parenthood. We have two frozen embryos left, so one day we will try for a sibling, but at the moment we are quite content with our baby boy, who will be here soon.

Looking back on our journey, I wish I'd known that there can be so many setbacks with IVF. I think it's so good to join an online community, to gain knowledge about all the paths you can take to become a mother. It gave me comfort that if IVF didn't work for us, there are so many ways you can become parents. Chatting with other men and women going through the same journey has been amazing and it has made us feel less alone. Even if it is reaching out to one complete stranger, it's nice to chat to someone who understands.

My favourite quote is: 'Don't measure your progress using someone else's ruler'.

Connect with me on Instagram: @ivf_got_this_uk

Chosen charity

Our charity is Miscarriage Association:
www.miscarriageassociation.org.uk

They offer support and information to those affected by miscarriage, ectopic pregnancy or molar pregnancy.

Alyssa

Alyssa and her husband live in San Francisco and have been trying to conceive since 2018. Alyssa shares more about their infertility journey, which includes one round of IVF, genetic testing, four embryo transfers, and the late loss of their son, Cole. They are still waiting for their rainbow baby.

Alyssa

My husband and I are both in our early 30s and live in San Francisco. We have always been eager to have children, both coming from large families with two siblings each. Having children, and having them soon, is something we bonded over very early on in our dating years. We actually started trying to conceive before our wedding!

When we first started trying, about three years ago now, we were so excited and hopeful. It didn't seem like a chore at all. I had been off the pill for a year at that point and we tracked my cycle using basal temperature.

However, our optimism quickly faded and after many, many months of loss, including the rupture and loss of my fallopian tube, we decided to see a specialist. In California, you have to be referred to one by your OB or you have the option of paying out of pocket to see someone of your choice. We chose to see an amazing and well-known doctor at a clinic that many friends and family members had used in the past.

We had known early on that my anatomy would cause some complications, but we were not prepared for what we were about to learn. I was diagnosed with Uterus Didelphis when I was in my late teens, which means I have two uteri and two cervices. After my tubal surgery, which happened on my right dominant side, the doctors had noted that my tube remained open and that we should be able to keep trying naturally.

However, my new RE ran a few tests and concluded that my tube was, in fact, closed. I was upset but happy to have a doctor I could trust and move forward with. My husband and I both eagerly signed the paperwork to start IVF. We were so hopeful and excited at that point. To be honest, we didn't even grieve the loss of being able to conceive naturally. We moved on quickly and counted down the days until our first shots.

At that point, none of our friends were actually trying to conceive or going through IVF. We were a bit in the dark but had family members to help guide us. We were very open with our journey from the beginning. We didn't have much shame around needing IVF to conceive and I wanted to make sure that our close friends and family were in the loop.

We started IVF in the spring of 2019. The process was overwhelming and confusing, but we quickly caught on to the stomach shots and crazy side effects that came with them. My body responded well to the medication and we were able to retrieve 24 mature eggs! After a week of growth, we were left with 17 beautiful embryos. We decided to do PGT-A (PGS) testing to ensure the embryos we were transferring were healthy. We felt it was the best way to set ourselves up for success. We were met with the amazing results of 12 PGT-A normal embryos! We couldn't believe it. We had 12 chances to build our dream family! We had eight boy embryos and four girl embryos.

After going through our initial IVF round, we let my body take a rest month. We travelled to New York and spent the week eating, drinking, and enjoying life 'just the two of us'. We thought for certain that would be our last trip as a family of two. When we returned from New York, we eagerly transferred our first embryo.

The doctor chose the embryo himself and it was a perfect, grade 5 hatching blast.

The FET cycle was much harder on us emotionally. I was so scared that it wouldn't work and my body wouldn't be able to carry a pregnancy. I had no idea what to expect and the medication the doctors gave me (progesterone and estrogen), made me feel pregnant and sick. I had to inject myself nightly in the glute muscle. This was hard and painful, but we got through it. I quickly learned what worked and what didn't work. When the time came to transfer the embryo, I had to be put under anaesthesia because of my anatomy, so I wasn't able to see the magical moment the embryo entered my uterus. My husband got to be beside me in the operating room, which was special enough for us.

The dreaded two-week wait is everything one would expect. You transfer an embryo then they send you home to wait. Hopefully, the embryo implants and begins to grow. However, this doesn't always happen. My clinic tests for beta (HCG in the blood), nine days after transfer. I remember that beta day. I had no idea what to expect. We don't test early, since it's important for us to wait for our doctor and the blood test, so we went into the beta appointment hopeful but realistic.

We got the call later that day and it worked! Our embryo stuck around! I didn't know the sex of the embryo, but my husband did and couldn't wait to surprise me. We then went in for our second beta, 48 hours later. I remember the nurse calling and telling us that unfortunately, the beta didn't double and I would have to come in for a third beta. This was the first time during that pregnancy that I was truly terrified of losing my baby. I had no idea what was to come.

Thankfully, the third beta was great and we moved on to schedule an ultrasound. I remember the fear that washed over me the first time I entered my RE's office for my ultrasound. At that point, I was so used to loss and bad news that I couldn't believe I was actually pregnant. So many thoughts go through your head once you're exposed to all that can go wrong. Will the baby be in my tube? Will the baby have a heartbeat? Will everything be okay? Thankfully, everything looked perfect. We got to hear little Peanut's heartbeat and it was truly a life changing moment. We had a viable pregnancy!

I was quickly brought back down to reality when my RE started talking to me about my anatomy. I have two uteri and the baby was in the right uterus. This added a whole new layer of complexity to the pregnancy. He told me I would be watched very closely and my expectations had been set, I was at risk for preterm labor. I was not to have sex, do high intensity workouts, or travel very far from my clinic or hospital.

We left our clinic that day and decided we would take our last trip as a family of two, down to the beach. It was far enough to feel like a vacation, but close enough that I knew I could be back at the hospital within hours. After that, we decided we would spend the entire pregnancy in San Francisco so that I could make my frequent appointments and be nearby if anything were to happen.

We graduated from our fertility clinic, hopeful and optimistic that our team of doctors at the hospital would be able to help us deliver our baby boy. I was quickly assigned a team of amazing doctors at UCSF. At that point in pregnancy, I was still scared to go on long walks, but I was starting to calm down a bit. When it came time to talk about prenatal testing, we opted in for all the testing that California offers, despite our embryo being PGT-A tested. We wanted to make sure our baby was okay.

Unfortunately, we received uncertain first and second trimester screener results, which completely threw us off. I remember being shaken when I received the call from the genetic counsellor after our first trimester screen results came in. Our little boy had 1:24 chance of having a specific syndrome. My placenta hormones were also off. Why, after all we had been through, couldn't this be easy? He was a PGT-A tested embryo. Didn't that mean he was okay? Unfortunately, most of the testing done isn't diagnostic and isn't always correct. However, we continued to push on and remain positive, hoping to get answers quickly.

Weeks 13-16 of pregnancy were a blur. I was constantly waiting for phone calls from my MFM (maternal fetal medicine) team. We decided to move forward with an amniocentesis. This diagnostic testing would remove some of the baby's DNA from my placenta and allow us to test for any genetic issues. We thought we were just being cautious and we were not prepared for the feat we were about to face. I was terrified for the amnio. I remember sitting in the room and squeezing my husband's hand as the needle went through my stomach and into my placenta. I was watching my baby on the screen the entire time, begging the doctor to please be careful. We got through the procedure. Everything was okay and the baby unharmed. We then had to wait a week for the results. I think that was one of my lowest points. I had no idea if this rainbow baby that we had fought so hard for was okay.

Being able to feel your baby inside of you is a beautiful thing, but when you're unsure if your baby is sick or not it becomes heart breaking. Some days, I would beg him to kick so I could feel him there, reminding me that he was real. Other days, I couldn't handle the little flutters. It was too hard. How was I supposed to live without my baby?

When I got the phone call that the amnio came back normal, I felt like I could finally breathe. It was as if the entire world was lifted from our shoulders. Our baby was safe inside of me. He would be joining us earthside.

We decided to announce our pregnancy at 17 weeks and we were elated. We lived in pure bliss that week. We had finally made it out of the darkness. We had professional photos taken for our announcement and proudly shouted it to everyone who would listen. I was pregnant with a boy! Many already knew about the pregnancy, and our hardships, but this was the first time we felt truly confident sharing the news with the greater public.

We started to discuss nursery plans, registry items, and names. I was almost 18 weeks and we had a lot to do! We had been holding our breath the entire pregnancy and could not accept that this baby was joining us. And soon! I was scheduled for a c-section at 35-36 weeks, due to my anatomy.

I started getting weekly cervical checks. I remember leaving for the first one on a Thursday and telling my husband, who had been there for every single appointment, that the baby was okay and it was just a cervical check. He could stay at work for this one. I walked into the room, eager to see my baby on the screen. I was 18 weeks along and could feel him dancing around. The tech started taking pictures and became quiet. An hour later, after taking dozens of pictures and unable to answer any questions I had, she told me to please call my husband and wait for the doctor. I immediately called my husband, who was able to rush over from work.

I'll never forget that day. We were at the hospital for seven hours. We talked to multiple specialists, including the Head of OBGYN. Our son was showing abnormalities on the ultrasound screen. They were fairly certain he would be okay with surgery, but they couldn't guarantee. There were medical books taken out, ultrasounds drawn on, words I had no idea the meaning of said, and many, many tears shed.

So, there we were again. Terrified that we were going to lose our baby. I had just started to truly connect with my son. I had bought him a few things for the nursery, announced to family and friends that he'd be joining the world in June, and had started to read to him at night. He was alive. He was moving. He HAD to be okay.

That day will forever be one of the worst days of my life. I felt helpless. I could see my baby moving around on the screen, I could feel him inside of me, but I couldn't help him. He seemed healthy to me. He was moving, so why wasn't he growing the way we had hoped?

From weeks 18 to 21 we did a variety of different tests. We did a fetal echocardiogram, a microarray, and an MRI. We met with the Head of OB, a pediatric surgeon, multiple MFMs, genetic counsellors, and my OB. To be honest, I don't remember much during those weeks. I just remember trying to remain hopeful and calm. At that point, we were just surviving. I would get up, head to the hospital, come home, try to eat, and then sleep. I had taken days and days off work because I was unable to concentrate. I just needed to get through it.

By week 22 of pregnancy a Whole Exome Gene Sequencing test confirmed our worst nightmare: we would lose our baby boy, Cole, to a rare genetic defect.

Our diagnosis was given on a Thursday in March 2020. We confirmed delivery for the following week. It was the very first week of lockdown here in San Francisco, due to COVID-19, and because of that, they couldn't confirm that my husband would be allowed in the room with me.

I remember sitting in the room, after seven hours with specialists that day, and hearing the genetic counsellor read us our report. To this day, it still feels like a dream. To be told your baby is sick and unable to grow truly crushes your soul. It changes your world. It throws you into a dazed shock that I'm not sure you ever truly come out of.

That Saturday, before Cole's delivery, I ended up in the Labor and Delivery emergency room. My anxiety had gotten to a point where I could no longer control it and I was diagnosed with Adjustment Disorder and heavily medicated. I honestly don't know how I made it through. I could feel my baby inside of me and it was heartbreaking. Why was the universe doing this to us? When you find out your baby is sick, especially so far along in pregnancy, your world forever changes. You get thrown into the unknown. A dark hole that is almost impossible to climb out of.

We had fought so hard for our son. So many years filled with procedures, surgeries, loss, shots, medications, and hope. We couldn't believe that our miracle baby was sick. That I had passed down a single gene defect that he happened to inherit.

On Friday, March 20th 2020, one week into the pandemic lockdown, we lost our son at 23 weeks. It was a multiple day process. My husband was able to be by my side the entire time, but we had to fight for it. Hours spent on the phone with some of the top hospital admin, trying to navigate how to make it possible. This pandemic was new for everyone and no one knew what to do. We were scared, overridden with grief, and in complete shock.

My medical team dilated me on the Wednesday, using a spinal tap and laminaria sticks. I was in Labor and Delivery the entire day. We went home that evening and enjoyed the last few hours with our baby boy. My husband had just started to feel him move only a few nights before. It was truly soul crushing.

On Friday morning, we went into Labor and Delivery. Almost fully dilated, I was ready. After some time, I was put to sleep, due to my body being in danger. I have a septum that was making it hard for me to deliver. My baby boy and I went to sleep at the same time and I woke up without him inside of me.

The first thing I asked when I woke up, was if I could see him. If he was okay. The doctor kept having to come in because I was so heavily medicated that I would forget we had already talked. The staff were so kind and patient. I can't even imagine what my husband's experience was, sitting in that delivery room beside me, watching it all unfold.

We named our son Cole. This name holds so much meaning behind it for us and we just knew it was perfect for our little guy. We had about an hour with Cole before we had to say goodbye. It will forever remain the most heartbreakingly beautiful moment of my life. We held him in our arms and cried. He will forever be our first born.

The weeks following the loss are still a blur. I could barely get out of bed. It's hard to navigate how to deal with postpartum without your baby, while also grieving his loss and being stuck at home during a pandemic. We were alone, unable to see family and friends, and my body was changing. We were in shock. It wasn't until my first postpartum period came, many weeks later, that I started to feel myself again. I started to gain hope and thought about trying again. Before then, I didn't know if I was going to survive. Most days, my husband had to make sure I got out of bed. I would collapse on the floor in his arms, unable to even move.

From the testing, we had learnt that I was a carrier of an X linked genetic defect that greatly impacted males. Thankfully, we were able to test for that genetic defect while I was still healing from the birth. By April, our remaining 11 embryos had been tested and we were given the news that seven of those embryos were healthy. This was the best news we had received in months. We had so much hope and that is what kept us going. Losing our baby was hard. It was, and is, probably the hardest thing we will ever have to go through as a couple. I just remember thinking, I am SO grateful for science and technology. Without it, we wouldn't have been able to identify Cole's defect. We wouldn't have been able to test our remaining embryos to ensure we, and our future children, didn't have to suffer a loss like that again. We wouldn't be where we are today, which is one step closer to a healthy pregnancy and baby.

After my second postpartum cycle, my RE said that we could try again. So, eager to be pregnant again with another little boy, we transferred another embryo in June. Looking back, I can't believe we tried so soon. I was still sick with grief and in total shock. However, I used the transfer as an excuse to pick myself up and move forward. I chose to transfer a little boy, in honour of Cole. I couldn't believe that I could possibly have another little boy so soon. However, the transfer failed and I was forced to take some more time off.

We then went on to do a hysteroscopy. We learned

that my lining was showing some trauma, which must have been from all of the medical procedures. I also have calcium deposits from Cole's birth. This news was hard for me to digest, but I allowed my body to rest.

Come November, we decided to try again. Another boy! At this point, I thought we were just still on the wrong side of statistics and that there was hope. We transferred our little guy and once again, the beta was negative. The only thing that got me through losing another boy, was the ability to jump right into another transfer cycle. Within days of my negative beta, I was doing shots again and planning our fourth transfer.

Our fourth transfer happened in December, and just a few days before Christmas, we learned that it failed. Again, another little boy lost. We soon realised, after three failed embryo transfers, that something needed to change. My body wasn't the same as it was when we transferred Cole. We decided to take some time away from IVF and heal.

My body is tired, but we remain hopeful. A break allowed us the space to focus on ourselves and our relationship. IVF and loss are hard. They test you. They test your emotional strength, physical strength, relationships, and mental capacity. I was broken for many months. I needed the space to heal.

We have recently jumped into another cycle. We'll be doing a test cycle, called an ERA, to run some diagnostic tests in hopes of pinpointing what's causing implantation failure. Depending on the results, we'll plan a transfer for spring 2021.

I am feeling hopeful, jaded, excited, and numb. After three losses and three failed transfers, it's hard to imagine things working out. The truth is, I'm not that terrified of it not working. I know how bad news feels at almost every stage – from implantation failure to second trimester loss. I know I can get through that. However, I am terrified of it actually working. I don't know what it feels like to go through a normal pregnancy. I don't know what it feels like for things to work out. We have four embryos left and our hearts are still full of hope.

My body, and our hearts, have been through the wringer. However, we're still full of hope and gratitude. I feel it's so important to keep pushing forward, keep reminding yourself that this fight will be worth it. And that, without IVF, many of us wouldn't even be able to make it this far. This journey has taught us so much. We have learnt to be resilient when we thought we couldn't carry on. We have learnt to be patient and let my body and our hearts heal. We have learnt how to be vulnerable and share our journey with the world, in hopes of helping others. We have learnt how to communicate better as a couple and how to work as a team against this unimaginable battle. We have learnt to pick ourselves up again, time after time, and remain hopeful. We have learnt that sometimes, parenthood doesn't mean you get to bring your baby home with you.

I'm hopeful that this next transfer will give us our rainbow baby. However, if it doesn't, we have a plan. And that is what is keeping me pushing forward. IVF is hard, loss is crippling, and dealing with it all during a pandemic is defeating, but we will keep pushing forward.

Connect with me on Instagram: @healthyivf

Chosen charity

Our charity is Resolve:
resolve.org

Resolve: The National Infertility Association is dedicated to ensuring all people challenged in their family building journey reach resolution through being empowered by knowledge, supported by community, united by advocacy, and inspired to act.

Keeley and John

After seven years of TTC, an initial diagnosis
of unexplained infertility, eight rounds of IVF with
Keeley's eggs (in three different countries), and
finally one round of IVF with donor eggs, they had
their little boy, Freddie, in June 2020.

Keeley

If you had told me a couple of years ago that our baby would be 'made' in Russia, it's likely I would have laughed at you. Not because I didn't know that doing IVF abroad wasn't an option, but as ever, you just don't think it's an option you need to consider… until you do.

First off, I'm a lucky girl, and am not ashamed to admit it or be proud of it (slightly, in a very nice understated and humble way). I live a very nice life. I had a pretty awesome childhood, was spoilt but in a very positive way, went to a great school which I loved, met amazing friends, went to Uni and met more amazing friends. I started climbing the career ladder from the bottom up, and worked at some amazing places that have made me the Producer I am. Met some more amazing and talented people, some of whom are my best friends today. Don't get me wrong, there has been a load of shit that goes along with all of that, but that's another story! (N.B. I love the word 'amazing'!).

I was single at the wrong time – i.e. my 30s – or rather, I hadn't really found the person I wanted to settle down with. My mum was starting to worry I would never find anyone to have a family with, as mums do. I also loved my career (although it has been brutal at times), but I've had some amazing experiences (some awful and stressful ones as well), so I just bumbled along. I never wanted to 'settle' and I am so glad I went through all of that, because it means I married Dwighty (my husband, that's not his first name). Despite the fact we went to school together (well, he's a toy boy), we didn't get together until 16 years later! He's my soulmate, and I couldn't have gone through all of this with anyone else…

So, I come to the point of the drivel above. I would never have settled, but I'm not going to lie, trying to be a mum in your mid-to-late 30s (40s!) is exhausting and no one tells you that might be the case (even though you sort of know it). I mean, because I'm the lucky one right, so why would trying to have a baby be any different? It should just happen, like everything else and to everyone else. Wrong… this is what happened, what I have learnt and what I am still learning. Eight failed IVF treatments, one natural pregnancy, one miscarriage, and one donor treatment later, we finally brought home our gorgeous little boy, Freddie, and every day is still a school day.

So here it is and what I have learnt:

It's ok to have a career and meet the love of your life later in life. I wouldn't have changed what I did up to the age of 33 for anything. Some of those experiences people can only dream of, and that was my life. Meeting and committing to the man of your dreams in your 30s is actually one of the most grown-up things I've ever done (not saying that meeting someone in your 20s isn't, by the way!). A little later in life, you just know what you want and what you don't, you also play less games. I think Dwighty and I knew it was forever from our first date, and that isn't an exaggeration. Ahhhh. We always knew we wanted a family – we told each other over a lychee martini – and being the healthy, active and kind people that we are, we just thought that was a given. As we have

89

discovered, that's not always the case.

We started trying about three months after getting married. I was 35 and already conscious of my age, and I knew it might not happen straight away, so hey, why not crack on? We kept trying. Less about the pee sticks, just more sex. Friends kept having kids, whom I love to pieces by the way, but it doesn't mean to say that when you see all your friends spawn out loads of kids between them and get pregnant by just thinking about it, you don't feel a teensy bit jealous and wish that was you… you do, every day.

After a year, we decided that we should go to the doctor and just make sure everything was ok – I mean nothing's a given. We went to the GP, and various blood tests etc later, we were told that everything was normal and they couldn't explain it. We had what is affectionately referred to as 'unexplained infertility'. At that point, we decided that IVF, or at least some form of assisted reproduction, might be the way forward, so we began the journey. Amazingly, we were informed that in our area of London, we qualified for three rounds of treatment on the NHS, so we started the process. However, it quickly became apparent that the wait times were lengthy – over a year before we would actually get treatment. The NHS were great, and our consultation was positive, but a year felt like forever, particularly for someone who didn't have time on their side as a geriatric mother! That's actually what they call you when you are a mother over 35… I mean, please?! We are very lucky that we could afford to, so we decided to head down the private route for treatment, because quite simply, we could start straightaway.

More tests. The same tests. More tests. HyCoSy – which checks the tubes are in working order by sticking a load of saline solution in your uterus. Intravaginal scans (repeatedly). Still 'unexplained infertility'…

So we go for it….

Although some of my close friends have had difficulty conceiving, and some have had drugs to help them along, none of them have had IVF. It's a strange old world and one that until you start talking about it, is a very mysterious one.

Once you start saying, 'We are going through IVF', it's amazing whose friend of a friend has been through it! Sometimes it helps, sometimes it doesn't, sometimes you are like, 'That's great, but I'm not them', and everyone has a different experience. It's a confusing and scientifically baffling process, but an incredibly humbling and amazing one. Once you start becoming an amateur expert on fertility, you realise how f**king difficult it is to conceive, and how anyone actually gets pregnant naturally in the first place is nigh on impossible! Injecting yourself, carrying around syringes and popping pills at odd times of day becomes weirdly normal. Disappearing into a room at work, or the bathroom, you start to actually feel a bit dirty, a bit like a hormone addict. You are a walking pharmacy. Blood tests are like buying a pint of milk from the shop – every other day, you pop in and then carry on your day like nothing has happened.

Our first round, although bizarre and slightly surreal, was a fairly straightforward process. I responded well to stimulation and we collected nine eggs, four of which fertilised. We had one put back in. Seeing your embryos up on a screen and having to identify them as yours is bizarre but kind of cool at the same time. That could be your baby and to all intents and purposes, I kind of think it is, even though it's just a collection of cells. You have the dreaded two-week wait… it didn't implant. Back to square one. We always knew IVF was never a given, but you do kind of hope it will just happen the first time. I mean, I'm lucky right? So naïve! I mean it happens, it does, but when the stat for conceiving through IVF is 1 in 4, someone has to be the other three!

Four months later we go again: same clinic, same process. Although I have to say, I wasn't in love with my consultant's bedside manner – you just believe they know what they're doing and you have to place your trust in them and go with it.

Blood tests, scans, blood tests, scans, injections, more injections.

I was lucky in some respects that the drugs didn't affect me too badly, although you would have to ask Dwighty to verify that! Collection, yeah eggs! Fertilisation, yeah three! One goes back in, on our wedding anniversary – must be a good omen. One of the worst experiences of my life. During transfer, they 'lost' the embryo. Never heard of that? Neither had we, and neither had a million other people that we spoke to after it happened, and neither really had the consultant! We were that 1% of cases something happens to… of course we were. They had transferred through the catheter (after having done a practice round, which they must do), but the consultant was having difficulty getting the catheter through. I have a retroverted uterus, which although makes it a little trickier, is not unusual and should never be a problem. So, she decided to change the catheter. The catheter and embryo went back to the lab, whilst I'm lying legs akimbo on the bed with a speculum in and Dwighty holding my hand.

10 minutes pass…

15 minutes…

Finally, the lovely nurse decided to make me more comfortable, i.e. take that bloody thing out of my vagina! Our consultant came back in. Now, when she first said this, we couldn't quite believe what she was saying. When they went to change catheter, they had LOST the embryo. What this means is that when they went to flush the catheter out, the embryo wasn't there, so it must be in my uterus, but they couldn't confirm! In theory, there was no other place it could be, but it wouldn't have been in the optimum place. We were in shock, and our after care was pretty shocking too. We sort of just walked out in a daze (my mum was there too, bless her). One minute we were hoping for our second chance and the next, nothing, just a 'lost chance'.

After about 24 hours, I then got really angry. How could this happen?! So we started complaining and trying to understand what went wrong. The consultant just said, 'These things can happen' and that was it. We changed consultants. We just felt so let down and there's no way we could trust her again.

More friends were having babies. Younger friends were having babies. Luckily, an amazing nurse there recommended another clinic, a total shift change, and it felt like what we needed.

More tests, blood tests, scans…

But this place was something else – a step up from where we had been, purely in terms of the intense nature of the treatment and feeling like they were throwing everything at you to make it happen. I started having immunology tests, to test my natural killer cells. Apparently my Cytokines (which are chemical messengers in the blood) have a tendency to elevate and I was given drugs to 'normalise' my levels. After two rounds of HUMIRA® (bizarrely an arthritic drug that does this), we were ready to go. Getting up at 6am to be in Harley Street for 7:30am blood tests every single day! IVF boot camp is what I lovingly referred to it as.

Having your phone on in every meeting at work, ready to take your instruction for drugs that day, going back two hours later for more tests or another scan. Waking up at 5am to do another injection, before the other four you have to do that day. Injecting in the meeting room. But again, I responded (not as well as the first two but I did respond), we collected three eggs and one fertilised.

The consultants were amazing, and despite our previous care, we trusted them implicitly. They had an irrefutable reputation, although it felt a little impersonal at times. You are a bit of a number, but if it gets results hey, who cares?! Having said that, there's one nurse there whom I trusted completely, and she was amazing at looking out for us. I think sometimes you just click with people.

Transfer was a dream (anything compared to last time), and we waited…

Anyone who's done it will know that that two-week wait is the longest two weeks of your life. The morning of the blood test, we walked for three hours, had breakfast and waited for the phone call. Three rounds and nothing, surely the third time should have been lucky, right? Wrong. 'Fourth time lucky' became our new mantra.

We'd had three rounds of IVF in 18 months.

All of the above was happening whilst I was working my arse off, with amazing support from friends, family and work, but anyone who works in advertising production knows that it is relentless, unforgiving, long unsociable hours and stressful (despite being fun!). I work hard, always have, can't not commit 150% all the time, and although people say that you should 'just relax' when you are doing IVF, or trying for a baby, are they f**king kidding! I mean you try, but… Although I have realised what stress can do, and that I have been stressed at periods over the years, and I know what people say about stress and pregnancy. We kind of realised that we had been doing everything possible to make the treatment work and it wasn't. Something had to change.

It was one of the most difficult, and yet one of the easiest, decisions I have ever made. I needed to try and eliminate any factor that was being detrimental to the process. So… I quit my job.

Although it was hard, I knew that after 17 years of working tirelessly, I hoped I had established myself enough for it not to make any difference when I decide to go back. For once, I had to put my personal life first and the time was right. I felt burnt out, both from the intensity of my job and everything we had been going through. It helps if you have amazing support. Dwighty didn't have to think twice about it, as he says, 'You just make it work'.

Lots of things go through your head during this process. You start to doubt yourself and blame yourself. It must be me. I must be the thing that's wrong (even if it's unexplained). Why is my body doing this to me? Why won't it work? You feel like a failure, even when everyone is telling you how amazing you are. For once, I wasn't trying to juggle a million things at once, I could concentrate on just looking after Dwighty and I.

Most people were really supportive of the decision. I did have a few people say: 'But won't that make it more stressful if that's all you are thinking about?' and 'You won't have anything to take your mind off it'. I can tell you: ABSOLUTELY NOT! For the first time in a long time, I put me first. I started properly exercising again (I've always played sport and been fit) and I started to feel like my old self. I always found it so difficult to find the time to go to the gym or train when I was working.

We have never 'eaten badly', but because I had the time to cook (not just grab a ready meal from M&S on the way home from work), we started eating even better. I love cooking, but I never did it, because I used to get home at silly o'clock and my fab husband was always there with dinner for me! I started changing just a few things, still eating the things we always had, but finding substitutes for others. Making my own protein bars (I know seriously, who am I?!)... I just found it really fun and interesting, finding these things out, experimenting and coming up with some delights... and a few disasters.

I also spent more time with my family. Seeing my mum for coffee and babysitting nieces and nephews, just being 'around' or 'present'... not checking my phone every five seconds, or 'just taking a call' during a meal out that lasted 45 minutes, while everyone has finished their dinner and are onto dessert.

Three months almost to the day after this kick starter, we were gearing up for another treatment (fourth). I had to do HUMIRA® again, twice (which is essentially a six-week process: two injections, two weeks apart and then a three-week wait for blood test and four days for results!). That week, I was waiting to come on my period, ready to start feeling like a human pin cushion again and...

WE FELL PREGNANT! NATURALLY!

A getaway weekend to the awesome San Sebastián did it, we think?! Bloody typical and true to every cliché in the book. Yup, will repeat that... we fell pregnant! Naturally!

I woke up, being three days late, and I'm never late. I had a test in the bathroom and just thought, 'I may as well, let's just check'. Three positive home tests later and a blood test at my clinic, I finally believed it. We were in shock, complete and utter shock, but elation at the same time... how could this have happened?

Then, by the way, you get a lot of people saying, 'Oh yeah, this happens all the time. You often find people having gone through IVF get pregnant naturally'. Well when it hasn't ever happened for you, those stories are great, but you kind of want to tell people to p*ss off. This isn't normal, because it's never happened TO ME!

You can imagine what the family was like (especially the mums), people were so delighted for us, but worrying nonetheless, trying not to get ahead of themselves.

It took a few days to sink in, but the realisation that we had fallen pregnant, that an embryo had implanted and that this was happening, was just the best news. The inherent anxiety of IVF, and the failures that have come before, are always there though. And it's us, right... the unluckiest conceivers in the world.

When you are in IVF, they scan you VERY early, like at 4-6 weeks... And they expect to see a gestational sac. My hormone (HCG) levels were very high, and they thought I should be further along, but my periods are very regular, so I said I couldn't be.

Having IVF and becoming knowledgeable about conception is great, but you also become far too aware of science, hormone levels, etc, etc. We know detail that anyone who falls pregnant naturally will never ever know about and would never doubt – sometimes it does your bloody head in!

The next rollercoaster began.

For the next week, we were diagnosed with a 'PUL' (yup a new term!) – a pregnancy of unknown location, no less. They couldn't find the blighter anywhere! We had new worries about ectopic pregnancy (could I lose a tube if that was to happen? God what would that do for our chances either way?!).

A night in A&E. Not that I had any symptoms of ectopic or miscarriage but the anxiety over what was happening was all consuming. We just wanted to see a doctor…

CHRIST ALIVE!

By this point, we had been referred by our clinic to our local EPU (Early Pregnancy Unit) at Whipps Cross (we are East Londoners!). We had seen them three times during that week, for more blood tests and scans. Of course!

Four consultants later, an amazing consultant stepped into our lives. She finally found a gestational sac – we are now 5.5-6 weeks pregnant. Another wave of relief, it's in the right place, it's there, she can even tell us where it implanted!

BUT (yup another one), it is very small for the stage that it should be at. Having discussed all of our history with her, her advice was to wait. Wait 2-3 weeks and see how it progresses. What's the harm? We've waited this long and it could happen. She didn't want to give false hope in any way but it could still be viable – outside chance, but a chance. We'll take that. So we wait. And wait.

It's a nice relief not to have blood tests or have various people looking at my vagina for two weeks, I tell you. Although you do develop an immunity in that regard.

Deep down, I knew it wasn't happening. From the day we saw her, I started to bleed, but only a little, so then the confusion of whether this is 'normal early pregnancy bleeding' and everyone you talk to says, 'Oh yeah, I had a bit of that, don't worry'. But I just knew. It's so hard, you so want to be positive, but when all you've had is disappointment, you protect yourself. I just knew.

We went back for our scan, and she confirmed that we have a 'possible failing pregnancy'. Because I've been on IVF drugs to support the baby, she says to stop and hopefully this will cause the pregnancy 'to pass' naturally.

Sure enough, three days later… it happened.

Not going to lie, it was not pretty, and sitting on a loo, crying, realising what is happening, is not fun. You go through emotions of what could have been, to thank god that it's over, to do I have to go through all this again? You are wiped out. BUT… I'm lucky. It could have been a lot worse, and although in no way am I trivialising this, I had sort of come to terms with what was happening before it happened.

People are still telling you you're amazing and brave, and that if anyone deserves a baby then it's you. They are right, we do deserve this, but I don't feel amazing and brave. I don't want to be amazing and brave… I want to be a mum.

Back to the IVF boot camp. And a lovely cocktail mix of the following, more or less every day:

• Fostimon® – which is a form of follicle stimulating hormone (FSH).

• Merional®   also used as part of the hormone treatment for stimulating ovaries. (FSH & LH)

• Cetrotide® – a synthetic form of a natural hormone that blocks ovulation. This prevents a premature surge of LH (Luteinising Hormone – which is the hormone that ultimately results in the release of the egg from the ovary) and allows the follicles to develop fully. This is the one they seem to believe you have to take at 5am!

• Aspirin – thins the blood and this can help in improving the blood flow to the lining of the uterus, which may help improve the chances of implantation.

• Clexane® – also helps to thin your blood and works by stopping blood clots forming and improving blood flow to the uterus and lining, and in turn helping with implantation. Anything sounds good!

• Levothyroxine – another little gem to help the whole process and my immunes. Thyroxine controls how much energy your body uses.

• Dexamethasone – a steroid and an effective way of treating inflammation in the body and this also may improve implantation. I'll take that, thank you!

• Cheeky course of antibiotics after my cyst aspiration, which gave me some lovely side effects that don't need to be elaborated upon!

Straightforward does still mean: Cetrotide® injection 5am; tablets in the morning before I leave the house; 7:30am blood test; Fostimon® / Merional® injections when they 'call' after my bloods have been screened (which could often be straight away, I was in the loo in John Lewis once!), and Clexane® 12 hours after my aspirin.

Another three rounds of all of this go by, and we still don't have our happy ending. Six rounds of hope and disappointment.

This isn't supposed to try and illicit any sympathy, by the way, it's more just to explain what is actually involved in the process, for those who might not be aware (well, at my clinic anyway, and mine is extreme) and every treatment is different and very personal, both to the person and to the clinic involved. I think it's really hard to understand if you haven't been through it, and that's not a slight on anyone as I wish we didn't have to, but I think it really is important for there to be an awareness around the commitment and the level of 'stuff' that is going on, whilst you are trying to 'relax' and 'not think about it too much'! And to hopefully explain why it's sometimes hard to keep this all to yourself and still continue living your 'normal life'. This process doesn't equate to normal, but it becomes your own sort of normal.

Dwighty has always wanted to be a dad, and the fact is, I knew he would make the most incredible dad, and I wanted that to start as soon as possible. But as the male in this process, I can only imagine the sense of helplessness that consumes them. Aside from making sure your 'boys' are in tip-top condition (and this is super important, believe me, it's not all the woman's body that contributes to this process working), what else can you do? Dwighty went along with my health kick recipes, my ban on 'refined sugar', protein with every meal, a fascinating array of quinoa variations and broccoli rice, alongside my militant approach to alcohol (although the odd IPA or shandy did creep in but hey, we are all human!). But, he did it because he knew that ultimately it was the best thing for both of us, physically and mentally, and also because doing it together was really important. You are in this together, and any elements that can make you feel closer to each other as part of the process is, in my opinion, really important.

I also think, 'God bless them'… do you know how embarrassing it is to provide 'a specimen' and then come out of a fairly uninspiring room (!), to a waiting room full of people, who all clearly know what you've just done? I mean, come on, that's excruciating! A slight dip of the head and take your seat. I'm under anaesthetic when I'm having my 'bits' collected, blissfully unaware, but there is something so cold about that little pot and that brown paper bag! Although, you do have to laugh about it, and we found that having a sense of humour about it all, and really trying to find the positive is so important.

The one thing I know is that Dwighty always wished he could just 'fix' this. He is amazing at 'fixing' things, whatever that might be: my inadequacy at general household technical maintenance, or him helping friends through tough times. Dwighty always knows exactly the right thing to say and do, but this isn't something he can fix on his own. And I think that's hard for anyone, but especially for blokes. But we are in it together and it is a partnership, and has only made me love him more (sorry I know, I know, but it's true). This doesn't always happen and can often really drive couples apart, which is so sad, but I can see why it's possible. It's brutal, unforgiving and more often than not, soul destroying.

Half of my friends were well out the other side of having young children, and I hadn't even begun. It's the old adage isn't it, and it's a terrible feeling, but I honestly just felt like we had been left behind. I always envisaged my friends and I's kids playing together, hanging out at weekends, going on great holidays together and it all working because we all had kids the same age. At some point, I had to change my perspective and think, 'Well, at this rate, and all things being well, at least we'll have great babysitters'.

I've seen this a lot, this concept of 'being left behind', and not always in relation to fertility. In a culture where we are constantly comparing our lives to others, I guess this feeling is inevitable, but it's not good for us. I think there is a fine line between being ambitious in whatever sphere you want to apply that to, and being wholly aware of exactly where you are and what you actually need. A very smart cookie of a friend of mine, who is also a counsellor, said that actually decade birthdays (whichever they might be), are often times when we pause and reflect on where we are or aren't, or thought we would be. Also, that as we age, we increasingly need to accept what we can't control and just be ok with that, rather than fighting it. God, that couldn't be truer than in fertility I think, and turning 40 felt like that for me.

After six rounds of unsuccessful IVF treatment in London, it was time to make a change. We are firm believers that if you keep putting the same things in, you get the same results, and it was time to change the variables. Obviously our treatments had been continually tweaked over the years, and that's not taking anything away from our clinic, but we just felt we had come to the end of that road. With the options in front of us, it felt like if we were going to consider different treatment options, then why not change it wholesale.

At the stage when we first went abroad to Spain, we were still using my eggs. We had looked at various tests that we hadn't yet done and having discovered that actually some of these originated in Spain, we thought why not just go straight to the source.

The change of environment was quite invigorating; the novelty of discovering a city was exciting, living like a local was quite empowering! Finding a new routine, a new way of being in a clinic was refreshing, having been used to a familiar protocol for so long. I know this can be unsettling for some, but I saw it as an opportunity, as a way of finding new hope.

Our consultants in Spain were great (admin not so

much), but they had a plan, and we love a plan! I'm a producer, so understanding the solutions available, creating a schedule, a plan and curating the best talent is what I know. The plan was that we collect and do PGS testing on any embryos created, given my run rate, we were looking at three or four more rounds to get enough numbers to test. Although it felt good, as we would know the viability and quality of the embryos, it also started to feel like we were climbing Everest again. On our first round in Spain, I only produced one or two follicles; luckily, they contained eggs and we managed to get one embryo to test… it came back abnormal. We went again six weeks later, same result… I didn't need to do any more rounds – I knew what the results would be and I was done. I was exhausted, but I also knew what our next step needed to be, and I wanted to take it. We needed to move on; we needed a different path to make our family.

I often get asked how I picked myself up after so many rounds of disappointment, and it's a hard one to answer. Everybody is different, so it will change how you reconcile and deal with each stage. I am generally a really positive person, as well as being pretty competitive, so I sort of refused to let all of this make me feel sad. I decided to try and take the positives out of every stage, and I just kept reminding myself that each step was a step closer to hopefully making our family, whatever way that ended up being. There are no guarantees, of course, but I knew I was doing everything in my power to try. If I'm honest, I think it also helped that I never had any extreme, indeed any really, physical side effects with any of my treatments. I didn't mind taking the drugs, I don't mind a scan, and I think because of that it enabled me to just keep going, because I knew I could cope with it. All of which I then took into donor treatment and our ninth round.

Moving to donor egg treatment wasn't an instant emotional decision process, although in the end, it was a fairly quick practical process (in the scheme of things) – from the end of PGS testing to picking a donor in Russia was about three months. In my head, this had been slowly happening for about a year, from around round four of treatment, as this was an option that had been broached then, and one that I thought might end up being our story. So, in my head I started to contemplate it, to understand how I might feel when this time came, which I inevitably thought it would. We had decided that if PGS testing came back abnormal, then it was our time to move on and find a different path. After eight rounds with my eggs, I felt we'd given it a bloody good go, and that I, especially, could find peace with that. We always wanted to exhaust the options before moving on, and we were lucky to be able to do that, but we also wanted to have a family, and time and my age did become factors. This timing is different for everyone. It's not a matter of how many rounds you've had or what the results of those were, it's not a competition to see who gave it the 'best go'! It's about what you want, your specific situation, and what you can process emotionally and financially.

Deciding on donor treatment isn't easy; it involves a lot of complex emotions. The acceptance of the loss of your genetics; the thoughts of the effects of your decision on your future child(ren); the debate around known and anonymous donors; the profile of those donors. Will I feel like the real mother? Will I bond with my child? How we will make this story theirs? etc… Then consequently, where you might want to make this happen brings a whole host of other factors and decisions – availability, wait lists, time, cost.

The way we narrowed down our options in terms of countries for donor treatment, was to really think about what we wanted to know about our donor. How much did we want to know? Did we want to know nothing at all? Did we want the clinic to take control of that process? Did we want to? What are the legalities in that country concerning disclosure at certain ages and the access to the donor? All these thoughts float through your head. Only you can make those decisions, and that will be right for you, no one else.

For us, we decided that actually, now that this option was our reality, we wanted to know as much as possible, but still have an anonymous donor. We also wanted to be able to see pictures of our donor as a child and know a little more about her – her motivations, her background, etc – and I wanted to feel that I had some affinity to that person, that I could feel or 'see' something in her that I recognised in myself.

This led us down two possible paths in terms of countries: the USA and Russia. We investigated both and decided on Russia. We'd never been there, would never have considered it, but now it felt like it was the most natural thing in the world. I think because it's so unfamiliar or unknown in comparison to the USA, it did feel strange to start with, but couldn't be further from the truth now. There was no need to be nervous about what to expect.

I had learnt of the clinic through an old friend of mine, and I knew from the first Skype™ call, and that first exchange of emails, that this might just be it. The most personable and friendly experience we could hope for. Super organised but highly approachable, and one of the best 'waiting room' and coffee machines we've had! Trust me, these things seem trivial but become important when you spend so much time in a place.

In contrast to previous treatments, this time it just felt different. On reflection, I now see part of this as a pressure that had been lifted from me. I didn't have to 'perform' any more, and I cannot tell you what a relief it was. It was all about the embryo, and I just had to give it the best home possible.

We explored St. Petersburg, immersed ourselves in the city and made the most of our time in the place. It is a beautiful city, which we are now privileged to have been to, and have a connection to forever. Yes, it was bizarre not being able to read or understand anything at all, to be so unfamiliar with day-to-day things, but actually this made it all the more exciting and a special part of what I think is now a rather wonderful story for us all. It was alien not to be visiting the clinic every day or indeed to be injecting myself, just a few patches and some tablets, how civilised! The day of egg collection was surreal – it was Dwighty's turn to be the star of the show, and I was there to support, to throw all the magic over it I could muster. When we knew that collection had been good and that all had fertilised, we went out and celebrated! We found a gorgeous restaurant, ordered some good wine and felt like this might just be our time.

Transfer day came, and this was the day we brought our little Freddie home with us. We didn't know that then of course, but as I walked out of the clinic, I had so much more hope than I had ever had over the last seven years. Seven years of waiting and hoping is a long time; I never thought we would still be in the same position all those years down the line. I'm not one for 'signs', but the next day, we walked to a new neighbourhood near our Airbnb, and on the bank on the side of the canal, someone had created two huge hearts in the leaves that had fallen. I looked at Dwighty and smiled. Maybe this time, just maybe…

In many ways it was harder to shift my mindset into believing that I had more chance than not of becoming pregnant. After experiencing so much disappointment, and constantly battling the most ridiculous odds and percentages, everything was in our favour. On our last round of treatment with my eggs, our percentage for success was around 2%, which at the time felt bonkers that we were even contemplating it. We had always tried to steer away from percentages, we always preferred to view it as 'a chance' and that was good enough for us. However, at some point you have to face the facts, and when you know that moving to donor eggs would give us 65-75% chance of success, you can't ignore the stats. The shift was real, and we allowed ourselves to really hope, to believe.

Ten days later, at six o'clock in the morning, I woke, turned to Dwighty and said, 'I need a wee'. He was like 'err ok', but then realised what it meant. The pregnancy test turned positive by the time I had managed to pull up my pants! I just walked back into the room with my hand over my mouth, crying. The room was still dark, but I didn't turn on the light, god knows why! I got back into bed, Dwighty shone his phone torch on the test and we both cried. Cried for all the years of trying, cried for all the loss we had endured, and cried for all the energy spent, but mostly, we just cried because we were unbelievably happy!

The day we told our family and closest friends was just incredible, and for the first time, I knew I was telling them something that was true, something that would happen – that we would bring our baby home this time, and that's exactly what we did. He just wouldn't be here if we hadn't taken the path we did, made the often hard decisions we did, and trusted in our feelings.

Freddie was born on 23rd June 2020, after a straightforward and fairly enjoyable pregnancy (thank god!), and a planned abdominal birth (C-section, to those who prefer)... what we didn't count on was it would be in the middle of a global pandemic, but that's another book! As soon as Freddie was handed to me, as soon as I first felt his little foot in my hand, there was just the most incredible feeling of love, and there's no doubt in my mind that he is my son. I made him, my blood runs through his veins, and I see my smile reflected in his. I firmly believe in the magic of epigenetics, and without a doubt, although he wasn't made with my egg, he is every part of me, I determined which elements made him him, and I'm pretty pleased with the results!

It's not how I envisaged my pregnancy, or indeed the first year of his life, but he's here, and that's all that really matters. It doesn't mean I don't feel cheated, or that I might never know what it's like to enjoy all of this in 'normal life', it's been hard, but amazing. I think there is so much pressure on those who have been through infertility and bring home their babies, that they aren't supposed to moan or be able to complain, and I think it's really unfair. Yes, I have everything I ever wanted, but I'm human and being a parent is hard, whichever way your child came to be in this world. And even more so when that coincides with a global crisis. Infertility never ever leaves you. I may have a baby, but I am still infertile. So yes, I have Freddie, but I still love a lunch and some more of those would have been nice, sitting with friends, with new friends getting to know each other and our little people. Yet in the same token, if times had been normal, I know I would never have had the same sort of time with Freddie – I would have had to share him more, and we would have been busy busy, because that's who we are. What I hope, and I guess deep down I know, is that hopefully he won't really remember these strange times, and I hope he doesn't have to see people wearing masks for much longer.

And now we are on another journey; it never ends! We are learning to be the best possible parents to Freddie every day and will continue to do so for the rest of our lives. We are learning how we will tell Freddie the story of how he came to be, which is so important, and something that hopefully he will be proud of. I'm so passionate about being open and honest, but also ensuring that it doesn't define him – it is just a small part of who he is and who he will be. We are learning how to make the best life possible for all of us, and what that looks like. Mostly, we are dreaming of the gorgeous little boy he will grow into, and already is. His giggle is infectious, he is the most placid, chilled and happy little boy, and as a result, I know we are doing at least something right.

When I think about how I feel these days, mostly I'm just thankful. Thankful for the miracle that science has given me; that it has given us the opportunity to be parents. That there exists in the world people who are willing to do incredible things for others. That infertility has both enriched and changed our lives irrevocably. Of course, sometimes you wish things had been different, but if they had been, we wouldn't have Freddie in our lives, and that just doesn't seem possible.

Connect with me on Instagram:
@_tryingtobeamum_

Chosen charity

Our charity is Fertility Network UK:
fertilitynetworkuk.org

They provide information, advice, support and understanding for those dealing with infertility.

Louise and Kevin

Four years trying to conceive. Three rounds of ICSI. One round in Belgium, with an add-on not available in the UK at the time, which resulted in a pregnancy but a missed miscarriage at nine weeks. Whilst deciding on their next steps, they conceived naturally, and their son was born in the summer of 2019.

Louise

There are certain moments from our 'journey' to have a baby that are burnt deeply into my memory forever:

1. My husband's face drained of its usual optimism (making him look both so young and so old) as our GP told us the results of his first sperm test.

2. The phone call during our first round of IVF, when they told us only one egg had fertilised.

3. The bluntness of the consultant who, after our first round of IVF, said our chances of having a baby were less than 10%.

4. The image of what should have been our ten-week-old baby without the heartbeat we had pinned all our hopes on.

5. The complete disbelief of realising we had fallen pregnant naturally, after being told it was physically impossible for us. The ensuing 10 pregnancy tests I took to check it was true.

The types of memories where you can recount every minute detail as if it happened in slow motion. That heavy feeling of time seeming to stop around you. The weight of the situation making your breath shallow and ineffective. For me, infertility was a long journey of waiting, with time passing painfully slowly then punctuated by these high stake, stomach churning, stress-inducing moments where everything was brought in to a focus I didn't want.

Writing this, I am extremely conscious that my story is one of those that I hated to hear when we were trying to build our family. That 'miracle' surprise pregnancy that happened just as we had given up hope. I really do apologise if my story is triggering to you and the stage of your journey you are on. I know it would have been to me at the time, but I hope it also tells the story that there is often a lot that can be done to treat or improve male factor infertility, and that a dire diagnosis does not always mean the end of the road.

I am not here to tell you it had anything to do with relaxing, or how stressed we were. We conceived naturally when I was in the depths of mourning a loss, when I was too scared and stressed to even consider our next steps. Plus, that would imply that infertility is controllable by the mind (this would never be said to someone experiencing another disease), as if it's something to be conquered, a battle to be 'won', as if we can do the 'right' thing and unlock the door to parenthood. I think ultimately, it just comes down to luck: good, bad, or f**king terrible luck.

We started trying for a baby straight after we got married. The first year started with hope and not really paying attention. But as the months started to stack up, we moved on to ovulation sticks, symptom spotting, increasingly manic googling to cutting out alcohol, caffeine and popping vitamins I'd never even heard of six months previously. The months started to follow a regular, depressing pattern: at first hopeful, then the agonising waiting, then the disappointment, then trying to build ourselves back up again. After the text book 'year of trying', we booked the doctor's appointment we had hoped we wouldn't need.

An unsympathetic and unprepared GP told us our initial results were basically dire – natural conception was impossible and we would need medical help to have a family. My husband's results were worse than we were expecting. We had a suspicion that we may struggle to conceive, as my husband had an undescended testicle as a child. But we were not prepared for how bad the results were – the GP asked for them to be repeated as she couldn't quite believe them. But after another week of waiting, it was confirmed there was no error – we were going to need some help.

The NHS urologist we were referred to was clearly coasting his way to retirement. He offered us no suggestions or hope that anything could be improved, and had no interest in any treatment for male infertility – just that ICSI was our only option and that it was expensive 'but so are children', so it will prepare us for them. Even as rookies, we knew it was a bad patient experience, with a complete lack of helpful advice or investigation, but we weren't to know for a couple of years and a lot of heartbreak later, just how outdated and plain wrong this advice was.

I remember thinking it seemed unfair that the treatment burden was falling solely on me and there was nothing available to try to improve my husband's situation. But as newbies to this world of acronyms and complex science, we put our trust in the specialists and accepted that IVF would be our route. After grieving the natural route not being an option for us (this was a real grief for both of us at the time), we entered our first round with optimism we were potentially starting a family.

We were incredibly lucky to get two free rounds on the NHS. And after months of waiting and endless jumping through bureaucratic hoops, it felt like we were finally making some progress. Our consultant at the NHS fertility clinic was positive and encouraging at our first appointment. She told us that as I was relatively young (32), we should get a decent amount of eggs and we should be able to build-up and freeze enough sperm for a round of ICSI – we had a good chance. But as she scanned me for the first time, I saw the concern flicker across her face, straining over the black and white images on screen. This would be an expression and a silence that would become the norm during our scans. She told us that my ovaries were very hard to find and that they were smaller and had less follicles than she would expect at my age. I could tell she regretted being so positive initially. She wished us luck as she sent us away clutching our paperwork, prescriptions and instructions, and I could tell she really thought we were going to need it.

We found the treatment surprisingly ok – I got used to the injections quickly and I had very few symptoms, so felt physically normal throughout. This lack of side effects turned out to be a warning sign, as we soon found out I wasn't really responding to the drugs. My ovaries were not playing ball – in fact, they were barely out of the locker room. Even after weeks of pumping them full of FSH, they remained small and unresponsive. At every scan, the sonographers scratched their heads, lamented that it was surprising given my age, and told us to prepare for getting very few eggs. We hadn't anticipated this part of the treatment not working and were already starting to realise that IVF may not be successful for us.

We entered egg retrieval day cautious and nervous, steeling ourselves for a poor outcome. I woke from the sedation, feeling hazy, but was instantly back in the room when I started to hear the doctors doing their rounds, telling everyone what their 'haul' was.

Through the flimsy curtains, I could tell other people were getting big numbers. I steeled myself even further for disappointment: 'Four would be ok; if we can at least get four we might be in with a chance'. But even that seemed like too many to hope for. When our turn came, I could have ripped the piece of paper from his hand as he slowly studied it: 'Well, you surprised us all and we got ten eggs'. Ten. Ten little chances. Ten! One might be our baby. We were surprised, thrilled, and really felt for the first time that this might work. We went home feeling buoyant. Relieved. Hopeful.

The call the next day came later in the day than we'd been expecting. I was stressed and anxious, but also thought if the worst had happened and we had no embryos at all, surely they would deliver that news swiftly and early on? The phone finally rang with the news of what had happened overnight to our ten chances: 'Only one egg fertilised. Five were immature. We don't understand what happened to the other four. I'm sorry, this is very rare for someone your age and with ICSI'. I still remember my voice cracking as I tried to respond. We asked what they thought may have happened, but they were stumped as to possible reasons – perhaps it was the eggs, perhaps it was the sperm, they just didn't know and there was no way of telling. So much of IVF remains a mystery; it is not surprising when the success rate is just 30% but when all your literal eggs are in this basket, realising so much is riding on old fashioned luck is a bitter pill to swallow.

We were advised to have a day 2 transfer, so we found ourselves back in the clinic the next day for our transfer. We tried to feel hope and excitement as we saw our little embryo and its magical flash of light on the screen, but we were both going through the motions, already bracing ourselves for this round to be unsuccessful. The two-week wait was long, drawn out and consisted of days filled with googling, symptom spotting and trying to control my emotions (impossible when you're on a concoction of powerful hormonal drugs). We dutifully waited to test, but my period came three days before we even made it to the official test day. That was it; round one done.

Our follow-up appointment was devoid of sugar coating: the consultant was negative and extremely down on our chances, telling us she thought we had less than 10% chance of IVF working for us. We felt like biological failures at 32, after just one round of IVF, and that our only way to have biological children was already slipping away from us. Writing this, I feel some anger, as this had a severe impact on my ability to trust my body, the process, or have any hope that things were going to work, and it undoubtedly made the rest of our treatment so much harder.

For our second round, we tried a shorter protocol, higher dosage of drugs and more monitoring. Unfortunately, things went much the same way: only one egg fertilised, we had a day 2 transfer, my period came before the end of the two-week wait. Our follow-up with another consultant was kinder, gentler and she was more interested in helping us look at potential avenues; she didn't think this should be the end of the road for us just yet. She also arranged for us to see another urologist – this time, one who was pioneering research in the field and would be able to see if anything else could be done.

So, that was our two NHS treatment rounds over. We were out on our own, into the world of private infertility treatment and didn't know where to turn. So of course, to the internet we went, and I found myself deep in the niche recesses of the online infertility world, where you can find people who have similar or rarer diagnoses or experiences. I met and spoke with other women who had experienced similar rounds and results to us. They had been told not much could be done but through tenacious research, they had improved their results drastically – in fact, many of them had gone on to conceive. These women and their partners had travelled across the Channel to Belgium, where they were using a new technique to increase fertilisation rates: Artificial Oocyte Activation (AOA), which helps overcome total or partial fertilisation failure. During a round of IVF/ICSI, the egg is placed in a chemical solution containing calcium ionophores, which can help 'activate' the egg and encourage fertilisation. It is important to state here that this is an 'add-on' and to proceed cautiously with any treatment add-ons, especially those with limited clinical trials. However, considering our results so far, the fact that a cycle in Belgium would be cheaper than in London, and we would have a nice mini-break in Ghent thrown into the mix, we decided we had little to lose.

Our consultant in Belgium was kind, understanding and passionate about the treatment and research she was undertaking. We felt cared for, listened to and like they would try all they could for us. They would test more throughout our cycle and I felt that the monitoring was more comprehensive, and the treatment more responsive, than anything we had in our NHS rounds. NHS treatment is wonderful (although it needs to be much more equitable) but from our experience, I believe it works best for those who respond in the 'normal' way. We felt that we were only offered one way of doing things and unfortunately, that didn't work for us.

We left beautiful Ghent feeling reassured and

hopeful, driving back to England with a boot full of syringes and drugs, like the lamest drug heist ever. We did most of our cycle at home, sending blood test and scan results back to Belgium, and when we got the go ahead that we were close to egg collection day, we headed over the Channel. We're lucky that we don't live a million miles away from the Channel Tunnel and could get there quickly; we didn't have to worry about perfectly timed flights. Although, we still found doing a cycle abroad taxing, and it added another level of gravity to the cycle and all we had riding on it.

We were happy to get seven eggs from our egg collection, but they told us from the outset that they weren't sure how many were mature. And so, the agonising wait for fertilisation figures began. We were more nervous than ever. The next morning went by without the promised phone call. I remember pacing Ghent's picturesque canals in tears, catastrophising that none of the eggs had fertilised, and this was the end of the road of us trying to have our biological children. That we'd come to a foreign clinic, tried this experimental treatment and even then, we couldn't get out of the starting blocks. It turned out the delay had been because they were unsure if some were going to fertilise and had been waiting to see what happened. The embryologist was tentative and nervous on the phone as she told us only three had fertilised. They were disappointed for us, they had expected more, but we were thrilled – three was such a huge improvement to us!

Now another wait started: the five days to get to blastocyst. We headed back to the UK, leaving our embryos hopefully doing their thing. Every day we held our breath, so far we had no idea if our embryos had ever made it past day two, but by the end of the week, we were thrilled to discover we had two embryos. On the morning we arrived back in Ghent, it turned out that only one looked good enough to transfer. So even with all the extra effort, we were down to all hope riding on this one little guy. Still, it was a blastocyst; it felt like the best chance we'd had so far. We quietly hoped this time might be different.

We headed in for the transfer and a doctor we hadn't seen before promptly gave us another large dose of harsh reality – she told us the blastocyst was dividing slowly and that there was a high chance of it either failing to implant or ending in miscarriage. The highs we had at the beginning of the week fell crashing down around us. Miscarriage was not something we had considered and it certainly wasn't something we wanted at the forefront of our minds as we had this precious embryo transferred back to us.

It was my husband's birthday, so after the embryo transfer we went to a depressing, out-of-season Belgian seaside town. It rained as we ate a soggy pizza in a tourist trap restaurant and we felt like we were in a sad romcom. We missed our Eurotunnel slot and sat in a daze whilst families coming back from holidays swirled around us. We got home and started another two-week wait. I tried to keep busy and knew I wouldn't test until the final day (I couldn't bear any more uncertainty), but was fully expecting for my period to come before that anyway. However, for once we made it to test day without my period putting a red dash all the way through our hopes.

So, test morning finally rolled around. I opened the test and could barely look at it as we waited. Miraculously, there was an actual line. The holy grail: a positive pregnancy test. We should have been thrilled; I am still sad we weren't. But we were too bruised and cautious to celebrate. The words 'high chance of a miscarriage' thronged through my head. We would be cautious, keep our heads together and wait to see what happened. Our clinic told us to book a seven-week scan and again, we waited patiently, yet increasingly nervously. I don't think for one day of those few weeks I allowed myself to believe it was a success. At the scan, I was a nervous wreck. I told the sonographer our whole medical history – the pressure on the poor girl must have been intense, but her face beamed as she moved the wand. She located a strong heartbeat and told us everything was measuring exactly as it should. We both burst into tears, from a mixture of intense relief and joy. Wow a baby, with a heartbeat! Our baby.

We were still in touch with our clinic and we spoke to our sweet, kind consultant. She was thrilled for us, and said the chances of a miscarriage at our age and after seeing a heartbeat were low. That she was very confident this pregnancy was going to progress, and we should now just see ourselves as a 'normal' pregnant couple. We told close friends and family, who were elated for us – they had been such an important part of our journey: cheerleading, supporting, and giving us space when we needed it. But I couldn't bring myself to be fully happy. I was scared, cautious, I still felt unsure of how things were going to end. Yet as the weeks went on and the blood that I checked for constantly never showed, I started to hope and think of an actual successful pregnancy.

We remained nervous, so booked another scan at just under nine weeks and to our relief, all was looking good – the flicker we had seen two weeks previously had turned into a little bean-shaped baby. But the reassurance from our scan didn't last long. I was still worried. I started to lose the hope. I didn't want to talk about the pregnancy, I would snap. Did I know? Or was I just protecting myself? Was I in a state of constantly being steeled for more disappointment? My worries continued to get louder and louder, so we organised another scan. We went into the same room, where three weeks before we'd had such joyous news. It was a swanky Harley Street clinic with large ultrasound screens everywhere. I still wonder about those screens, which must have displayed so much joy but also such sadness for others – why aren't they turned off until they know everything is ok? It was so obvious from the moment the cold probe moved across my stomach and the image appeared large on the wall, that our baby wasn't alive anymore. It was too small – the same size we had seen during the last scan. There was no heartbeat. It was still. It was gone.

The sonographer was kind, and left us alone with a box of tissues to try and compose ourselves, before we had to go back to the reception full of pregnant women to pay for the scan. Along with those big screens, I wonder why they don't get you to pay before. It seemed like a final dagger, this walk of shame like no other. I was on autopilot whilst my husband cried. We went out into the street and stood on the same steps in silence, where weeks before we had hugged and jumped up and down with joy at the good news of the heartbeat.

As the baby had grown to a decent size, I was advised to have a D&C, and there was no way I could have dealt with a contracted wait for things to 'pass'. We waited in an awful limbo, knowing the baby was still there, but also, completely gone. A few days later, the procedure was done. The nurses were kind; the consultant less so. He told me it was a good sign I had gotten pregnant and that four years wasn't that long to try for a baby. It didn't feel good; it felt terrible. We went home and I hid away. We isolated ourselves. We didn't know what we were going to do. I was extremely down – three rounds of ICSI in a row, all with disappointing results, had left me with no confidence in my body, and now I doubted my body's ability to maintain a pregnancy.

We knew we couldn't just do another round without looking at different options or changing something. The thought of another miscarriage being the result of more draining treatment felt like it might break me. But we also knew we weren't ready to stop completely. We decided to see a fertility nutritionist to rebuild ourselves a bit – both our fertility and general health. We also booked to see a urologist privately. It was clear my body didn't respond well to IVF, so we wanted to make sure there was nothing more that could be done to improve my husband's situation. At the same time, our long-awaited, second NHS urologist appointment came through.

Well, it turned out these two amazing urologists thought there was plenty that could be done. The appointments we had with both could not have been further from our original experience – not only did they have suggestions; they were confident there would be improvements. For the first time, there were options open to us and they didn't all fall on me. My husband had a varicocele repair, which is not routinely checked and fixed for men suffering from infertility, but there is emerging evidence that varicocele treatment will increase natural pregnancy rates and live birth rates. He was also prescribed Clomid® – a simple, cheap drug, which again is not the norm in male factor treatment.

The urologists thought it most likely that we would still need IVF, but that we would have done absolutely everything possible to maximise our chances and hopefully avoid another miscarriage. Of course, there was no certainty (there never is with fertility treatment) but this felt different. We were told that the treatment would take a few months before they would expect any improvements. We were starting to feel more hopeful – although I was still too scared to start to consider another round of IVF. I needed a long break and time to rebuild. I'd miscarried in June and we spent a very sad summer grieving our loss, trying to regain some of myself that had been lost in the constant googling, researching, worrying and stress. I saw a counsellor, who helped me focus on the here and now, which so often gets sacrificed in the always looking and thinking ahead during fertility treatment.

In the September, I realised my period was late. I felt like a fraud buying a pregnancy test, but I thought I would take one to stop me wondering 'what if' until my period arrived. But there it was: a line. A positive pregnancy test. I told myself it was faint; I couldn't trust it. It must be a chemical pregnancy. We were still hard wired for disappointment at this stage. We decided we would test again in the morning, so after a restless night, I tested again at about 4am. There was undoubtedly a line and it was darker. This routine continued – sleep, test, repeat – and I lined them up over the course of several days, studying the darkness of each line as if they would reveal the fate of this pregnancy, like ancient runes. At the end of the week, we had done 10 of the things! We were pregnant!

I continued seeing the counsellor throughout the early stages of my pregnancy, who helped keep me in the present and helped me to avoid spiralling into too much worry, but it was hard. I think I just have to accept that pregnancy is a stressful and worrying time for me, as it is for many women who have suffered loss or who have struggled to conceive. After a missed miscarriage, I just didn't feel I could trust my body or feel confident that everything was going to be ok. The 'scanxiety' was awful; we got quite a few private scans and the reassurance would last for a day or so, but then the worry would come back. It wasn't until about 20 weeks that we allowed ourselves to really believe it was happening. And gradually, as I started to feel the baby move, I was more and more reassured. We both later admitted that even until the moment our son was born, and we heard him cry, we hadn't allowed ourselves to fully believe everything was going to be ok.

Our son arrived in June 2019 and true to form, after making us wait for four years, he was two weeks overdue and labour lasted over 40 hours. He's worth every moment we waited for him; he has brought unbelievable amounts of joy and love into our lives. He saved us in many ways, his sunshine soul has healed us, and I will never not marvel at the miracle of him being here. It's hard to know how infertility affects what kind of parent you become. I worried I would be overprotective or full of anxiety, but I think we are probably the parents we would have always been. However, we certainly have an extra dose of gratitude and even in the more challenging parenting times, I know we will never forget how extremely lucky we are to be parents to this angel boy of ours.

Fertility treatment and our miscarriage has certainly changed me. I'm more vulnerable than I was before but have gained a steely resilience too. There's a comfort in knowing that as a couple, we can handle hard and sad things that will get thrown our way and we can rebuild ourselves. I still wonder exactly what made the difference to us, but I don't think we will ever know for sure. Undoubtedly, the urologists we saw and the treatment they recommended made such a huge difference and completely changed our chances. It remains so unjust to me that infertility patients must advocate for themselves so much, whilst they are in such an emotionally fragile state. It was only through getting second and third opinions that our path changed so drastically – we should have been given this chance from the very beginning.

These amazing urologists who are pioneering research into male infertility are rare – most professionals working in the infertility industry are gynaecologists, and the focus is on treating female bodies. Even though male factor infertility causes half of the issues in couples who cannot conceive, treatment for MFI has been systematically overlooked and ignored, as IVF is seen as a solution that circumvents male issues. But this is often not the case and puts women's bodies at the mercy of invasive, and often unnecessary, treatment whilst ignoring the root cause of the issues. This burden on women's bodies must be lightened – yes, IVF is a wonderful, medical marvel in many cases, but women's bodies should not be subjected to invasive procedures when treatment would be better directed at improving their partner's fertility. There must be equality for anyone seeking treatment to improve their fertility, the burden cannot fall solely on one half of the population.

Chosen charity

Our charity is The Chris Aked Foundation:
www.chrisakedfoundation.co.uk

They provide support to the children of families

dealing with cancer and other life-affecting illnesses, offering help through memory-making days, activities and counselling.

Marie

After experiencing sexual abuse at a young age,
Marie found out years later that it had caused
irreparable damage and infertility. She spent years in
pain before being diagnosed with adenomyosis, as
well as other chronic conditions, and has been through
multiple surgeries. Marie and her husband have been
trying to conceive for several years and, after an
unsuccessful round of IVF in 2016, are currently
undergoing multiple egg collections in the hope
of a 2021 transfer.

Marie

My name is Marie. I am 38 years young and I work as a clinician, both in the NHS and privately. I was born and raised in London. I am mixed race. I have had multiple gynaecological conditions surgically corrected. Currently, I have adenomyosis and an adenomyoma, and I have recently restarted my IVF journey. I am an incredibly private person; I always have been. I had never been on social media so it was a learning curve being on Instagram. I joined to learn about other people's stories, and I found myself entering an amazing world of support – something I was not expecting but something I needed, especially from other women.

Sharing my story is something I never thought I would do, but today I decided to share something difficult, in the hope that I can be a light for someone else. I know one day my husband might read this and I have no doubt that some of the issues in my story may upset some readers. I do not tell my story for pity. My journey up to now would not make sense without me sharing my experiences honestly. I have decided to remain relatively anonymous but my desire to help others in my position is far greater than some embarrassment I may or may not experience from telling my story.

Before I start sharing my experiences in TTC and you read my medical history, I feel it is important to disclose that my internal stress levels throughout my life have been extremely high. I am externally calm faced, any stress I might hold manifests inside me, like a knot tightening inside my belly. I faced many challenges as a child, which had irreversible consequences on my health. I was sexually abused from the age of 7 until I was 11 years old, by a family friend. Looking back, what happened is sad – I do not dwell on it, it is something that happened and where I am today in my life is miraculous. My own family are not aware of what happened, I have never told them. I came from a stable home life; you could say that my parents took their eyes off the ball.

I believe now we live in a time where we are still learning about sexual abuse, but over 30 years ago, there was extraordinarily little understanding of child grooming. In recent times, especially with the #metoo movement, we are more aware of the issue of people using manipulation and their power to silence their victims. My family are kind, welcoming and charitable. I am still to this day, despite everything, a gentle soul so it was no surprise that between my parents being trusting by nature and my fear of not wanting to worry anyone, this enabled the abuser for many years. Victims of sexual abuse live in secrecy, with unfair stigma and crippling shame, and I would not want someone who has been through any kind of sexual abuse to not feel good enough to be a mother. I did not have the choice as a child when I was abused. Now I have a choice; to be the voice of my story, my own ending. There is hope and I want people to know that. I would love to point out that I am an eternally happy soul. If you see me (even under my mask during a pandemic), I am most likely smiling. I have had many moments of pure happiness as a child and as an adult. I feel incredibly lucky to be here; I have so much love in my heart. I am a success story, no matter how my TTC journey turns out, although being a mother is something I know I would excel at.

Over many years, I have often thought about what kind of mother I would be. I have considered every detail – from where I would want to live if I have a child, the school I would like my child to attend, if my baby had a medical condition, if I'd sing to them the old French songs my dad sung to me? I have thought about and played through my mind every difficult conversation and scenario I could have with my child, and what became crystal clear is that the love I would have for them would be beautifully unconditional.

My journey starts here. I met my husband when I was 24. I was still studying, so we married when I turned 29 and I thought I had all the time in the world to have children. I had never met anyone who'd told me they were infertile; I'd never thought about it. I later met my reflexologist when I was 35 years old. I honestly did not know how my lady bits worked. She explained everything to me in a way that felt amazing and I think sparks were flying around my head with all the revelations. I realised that I knew nothing about fertility, periods, pregnancy, gynaecological anatomy, and infertility. I admit, I was completely clueless, and it is because I was never taught about those things, not in school nor at home. I am embarrassed to admit that. I genuinely believed fertility was something I didn't need to worry about. My extended family is big, and there is an assumption that women of colour are fertile.

Throughout my twenties and thirties I worked, I studied, I built a life for myself, my husband and I travelled – yes, I was in pain, but I genuinely thought I had time to have children and that when the time came,

I certainly did not think I would have any problems conceiving a baby.

One day, when I was 22 years old, I mentioned to an older female work colleague that I felt unwell and her response to me was: 'You are not special; everyone has their periods, and this is what it is'. My immediate thought was, 'Wow, every woman goes through this? That is awful!'. Knowing this, I decided to fight through it. On the days I was crawling on the floor in 10/10 pain, I repeated to myself: 'Everyone goes through this; everyone goes through this'. Unbeknown to me, I had multiple fibroids in my twenties, I had stage 4 endometriosis, blocked fallopian tubes and ovarian cysts. It would take another 14 years to get a diagnosis. These things made me extremely unwell, however I learnt to live with it, using painkillers when I needed to.

Just to give you a description of myself, I have brown skin and I've always looked quite young, which meant very often I was not taken seriously. I saw a GP for back pain when I was 24 years old and she said to me, 'Do you work as a cleaner?' – this was my first experience of discrimination. At that time, I was studying and decided not to pursue my back pain any further.

When I moved from London to the South Coast of the UK, I decided to see a doctor. I was 26 years old and struggling with painful periods. I was given the pill, which I had never been on previously. The pill caused extreme lows in my mood, which were scary. I mentioned this to the GP and she changed the pill, only for the same thing to happen. At that point, I said to myself, 'Well, if this is the answer, I prefer to stay as I am' – I did not want to add more things to my plate to deal with. I did return to my GP when I was 27 and I received a referral for a scan. It was to be my first transvaginal scan experience. I was scanned by two men; it was painful and traumatic. I left the practice with a severe migraine, unable to walk. I chased up the results from my scan a few weeks later, where I was told very casually that I had fibroids. The GP admitted to knowing nothing about fibroids. He printed off a document for me from Google and said he would refer me to a gynaecologist.

I was quite upset as I could have used Dr Google myself and I had no clue what it meant to have fibroids. My referral came through for a female gynaecologist. I felt hopeful and I thought I would be treated well and that she would be empathetic. From the moment I met her, I felt that she wasn't taking me seriously, nor was she listening. She made me feel like whatever was happening to me was in my head. She mentioned that my results from the scan carried out by the two men were lost and she laughed. She preferred to do her own scan, which terrified me. The gynaecologist gave me a sample pot to do a urine test in and said that after I'd filled the pot, to take it to the lab myself. The nurse who was in the room was horrified at the way I was treated and after the appointment, she apologised to me and kindly took my urine sample and sent it to the lab.

Every awful situation looks better with hindsight – I should have spoken up for myself, I should have done this or that. Looking back, this is what years of abuse does, it teaches you to become silent. I did not want to cause any issues and I didn't want to worry anyone. When I learned that black women in the UK are five times more likely to die in childbirth, I could not comprehend how that could be possible. My experience with a dismissive female gynaecologist was an eye opener and I knew I had to start advocating for myself;

I had to start speaking up. I was 27 but I looked years younger, I was alone, out of my comfort zone, extremely vulnerable and being treated terribly. I had so much to learn about asking for help and using my voice. I decided there and then that I was not going to go back for a scan with this gynaecologist and I never returned. Another year passed and the pains in my womb and around my belly worsened.

Eventually, on New Year's Day, I ended up in A&E in London with unbearable pains. I was asked to do a urine test to check for a pregnancy and the doctor on duty felt my stomach. I was told nothing was wrong with me and to take paracetamol and to go home. At this stage, my belly was huge – big enough that people were giving up their seats for me on the London underground (I never took the seat). When my clothes stopped fitting me, I started buying maternity dresses and tops.

I was 33 years old when I paid to see a gynaecologist privately, I knew something did not feel right. The gynaecologist wasn't able to scan me on the day. I remember him trying and I was a nightmare – he was very patient and kind, but I had just had too many bad experiences which led to me not feeling at ease with him. He decided to do a hysteroscopy under a general anaesthesia, which showed that I had a 20cm fibroid. I remember the consultant saying that the fibroid was the size of a melon. I also had other fibroids of various sizes pressing on my organs.

Perhaps now there are more minimal surgery options available for large fibroids, however at the time, the option for me was to have open surgery (open myomectomy) via the NHS. I was given a monthly injection called Zoladex® for six months before the operation. Zoladex® is a hormone-based treatment which lowers oestrogen in the body. The aim was to reduce my oestrogen levels to restrict any further growth of my fibroids and thin the lining of my womb before surgery. I was given Zoladex® as an injection every 28 days. A nurse or doctor administers the injection, which is inserted under the skin near the belly button. Being on Zoladex® gave me a much-needed break before my big operation. I had no periods during that time, however I did experience hot flushes and weight gain. I could live with those things.

After my six months on Zoladex®, surgery went ahead with the NHS. During this surgery, the gynaecologist could see that I had multiple issues with endometriosis, ovarian cysts and my tubes were blocked. The surgeon removed the fibroids and some endometriosis. A year later, in 2016, I was forwarded and approved for an NHS IVF cycle. The criteria was strict – from weight, to checking my breathing. At the time, I also fell into the age range of under 35 for the NHS Clinical Commissioning Group (CCG) in my local area. I walked through every process as if I were wearing a blindfold. I had no idea what I was doing but I carried on moving forward.

I completed one egg collection and one fresh transfer with the NHS. I had no idea what IVF was. This was 2016 – there were some online forums, but no Instagram for support that I was aware of and I had not met anyone else who'd gone through IVF. I just thought it was a sure thing – you did it and it worked. I went on what I would describe as 'automatic mode'. I attended appointments, injected myself as instructed and I let the doctors, nurses and embryologists guide the IVF. I also thought perhaps IVF was not something people openly talked about and so I decided to keep everything to myself.

Throughout the initial process of blood tests and consultations, the doctors were speaking to me as if I knew what was wrong with me. I had a strong feeling that I was being blamed for being in the position I was in, and some of those appointments were mortifying. I honestly felt so dirty that both my fallopian tubes were so blocked. The doctors kept repeating that I 'must have caught an infection at some point'. It's easy to say, 'Well, she must have known something'. It was up there with one of the worst experiences of my life. My husband was sat next to me and the doctor in the IVF clinic just kept reading off a sheet of paper with no eye contact. Without warning, memories I had left behind were laid out on the table in front of me, and I had to deal with it. I just did not know how I was going to do that – how was I going to speak to my husband? As we left the clinic, my husband said to me, 'Don't worry, these things happen' and all I can describe is that I felt myself drowning in shame.

I had completed the stimulation process, had my eggs collected and by day five, I was in significant pain. I did not have a clue what was happening; however, a fresh transfer was advised. The pain I was in on transfer day was like nothing I had previously experienced. I had to sign a document and I could barely hold the pen. I remember not being able to sit in the chair as the consultant explained which embryos they would use. Out of the eight eggs collected, five fertilised, two of my best embryos were transferred and my remaining three embryos from the cycle would be frozen. My bladder was full, as required for a transfer, but I had to empty it as holding it was impossible. I was in the worst mental and physical state. There were five people in the room during my transfer, including a male student – I just was not ready for any of this. I was operating 100%

on auto mode.

Anyone who has been through a two-week wait will tell you how difficult it is. My TWW was brutal. I cried and held my belly, talking to the embryos inside of me, begging for them to stick. I was in such a bad place. I was exhausted; I was confused. I had no idea that it would be a good idea to make plans during a TWW instead of becoming anxious. When my transfers failed to work, I was bleeding heavily, and I felt like this would kill me. The physical pain was frightening. My husband rang the IVF clinic who said, 'Sorry, it doesn't seem to have worked but you still need to come in for the blood test'. I felt like they just had to get through their tick box system; there was zero compassion.

I took pain killers, and I don't know how I got through that time. It was mostly just a sad situation. I went into the hospital for the required blood test and no surprise, I was not pregnant. I was so sick after the failed transfer. I remember being curled up in a ball on the floor all night, searching on my phone for a gynaecologist who could tell me what was happening. I came across a renowned gynaecologist, booked an appointment and drove three hours to see him. I had an MRI and he told me I had adenomyosis – which is a condition where the inner lining of the uterus breaks through the muscle wall of the uterus. It was the first time I had heard this word. Admittedly, at this time, the pain was so severe I felt like my life was not worth living. I broke down in the clinic, in front of the gynaecologist, something I have never done in my life, but for whatever reason that day I could not see a future for myself. The gynaecologist advised a hysterectomy. I was emotionally and physically drained, but I knew a hysterectomy was out of the question for me. I needed a break.

Two months after I learnt I had adenomyosis, I decided to take a trip to Thailand. I was in pain but continued training in Thai boxing – it felt good to be active again and I started to feel more like myself. It was in Thailand, four months after my failed transfer, that I received the news that my sister-in-law was pregnant. Immediately, when I received the news, I cried for 24 hours nonstop. The tears just kept rolling and my own reaction shocked me. I felt that it was not about my sister-in-law becoming pregnant but a delayed response to losing my embryos. I needed a time out. My emotional, physical and spiritual tanks were empty. There was also some resentment in me that I had been through so much. I returned home from Thailand feeling like something was not right. I came across an Ayurvedic detox called Panchakarma in Kerala and I took the solo trip to India for four weeks. I had never visited India before, but I think at the time, I was trying to anchor myself.

Overall, the detox was a difficult experience. However, during my time there, I was assigned two nurses and they showered me with their love. I have never received such care from women; it was a motherly love and we all got on so well. On that trip I met women who were recovering from cancer and women who had experienced multiple miscarriages. During my final treatment with my nurses, one of them prayed that I would one day have a child of my own. I have never been treated so beautifully. It was a trip that was good for my soul. I cried when I left, leaving behind so many amazing women. Taking a trip, even locally, is something I would recommend doing – getting out in nature and reconnecting with the beauty around us can be a healing experience.

I was completely oblivious to the fact that I did not

process the loss of my two embryos. I lost them and any mental support was non-existent. I have always been so strong, especially for others, that I ignored processing and recognising my own grief. Some months after my time in India, I visited my cousin, who took me somewhere beautiful on the island where my family are from and it just happened that there was a basket of names for unborn babies. I wrote down the names of my two embryos and put them in the basket, and that did something for me, it helped me to move on.

After my unsuccessful IVF, I decided to leave the South Coast of the UK and move back closer to London. I loved living by the ocean, but I wanted to come back and be closer to the city I love. I needed to start advocating for myself and after all my online researching, I found an OBGYN consultant with an expertise in miscarriage (one of a handful in the UK) and he pointed me in the direction of a consultant gynaecologist with a special interest in minimally invasive surgery. I was nervous to meet him, even so, I knew I had to get checked out.

Any nerves I had disappeared after my first consultation with my now-gynaecologist. Scans revealed that I had many fibroids, ovarian cysts, endometriosis and blocked fallopian tubes. In 2017, I was booked in for surgery. Although I'd had fibroids removed in 2015, by 2017 many had returned. Both my fallopian tubes were removed, as I was advised by my clinic that this could improve my chances of falling pregnant with IVF. I finally found a gynaecologist who understood and listened to me. He gave me the space to talk about preserving my fertility and because of what I said to him, he did not speak the word 'hysterectomy'. I respect that gynaecological pain is often so severe and many women must make that difficult decision, or often they have no choice, to have their womb removed. I know that I too will have to make that decision one day.

When I recovered from the operation, I could not face IVF. I had zero pain and wanted a life. I decided to take a break. I had three frozen embryos and that was my security blanket. The trauma from my first IVF cycle was more severe than I had realised and so, at the beginning of 2018, I reached out for help with a talking therapist (counsellor). It ended up being two years of talking and listening. Two years of hard work, where I slowly started to understand that nothing was my fault. I blamed myself for so many things and that needed to stop.

I remember seeing my gynaecologist and trying to explain my two-year sabbatical to him! I felt I was letting him down; he'd done this phenomenal long operation so I could try to have children and I was not ready. In my counselling sessions, some heavy things came up and I knew I had to deal with them for the first time in 35 years. It was a slow process, where the penny kept dropping. It takes time to see results from counselling. Finding the right counsellor was something I put research in to. I tried one other counsellor before finding the perfect fit for me, someone I could be honest and comfortable with and someone who could think outside the box. Counselling is invaluable and it is for everyone. Many of us learn to live with bad memories and pick up poor coping strategies, which end up becoming more damaging, not only for ourselves but for those around us too. I would recommend seeking out help to learn better ways to manage traumatic experiences. In my sessions, I have explored areas such as motherhood, well-being and having compassion for 7-year-old Marie. The first year of therapy was the most difficult. I was often left exhausted after sessions. I relived some painful times in my life. I had never fully understood what had happened to me. When my counsellor told me that what happened to me was wrong, I felt I could exhale. Finally, I realised that I didn't have to carry the weight of my past on my own. I have often thought, 'Did I waste two years where I should have been doing IVF?'. When I look back over those two years, they were well spent. I was pain free (the most pain free I'd been in twenty years) and because of that time my gynaecologist bought me, I was able to figure a lot of things out.

I believe that anyone who has suffered any kind of trauma or sexual abuse should seek out help before or during IVF. I was unaware of how taxing IVF is. It is an all-consuming, full-time job and if you have experienced trauma, you may need extra support to get through what is a rollercoaster of emotions. In IVF, there are many ups and downs. Most clinics in the UK will give their patients access to a counsellor who understands the IVF process.

I found a counsellor who specialised in childhood sexual abuse and because of her, I was able to process that day in the NHS IVF clinic, when the doctor told me things about my history that I was not aware of. I'd never told my husband about my history of sexual abuse, which as I write it now, seems crazy. It is difficult to explain this, but shame makes you hide a part of yourself from others. The thought of talking about the abuse just did not seem worth it for me. This is a good example of trying to shut Pandora's box, only you cannot; it's too late, it's been opened. The doctor opened my Pandora's box, and I did not even know what I was trying to hide.

I believe that during IVF, things you perhaps did not think were important can start to surface, or sometimes problems are magnified because the whole process can be stressful. Whatever challenges anyone going through IVF faces, I believe dealing with them and getting support is important, so emotions do not spiral. I spoke to my husband about the abuse and he did not have one ounce of judgement in his body, he just held me and cried. My whole thinking in not telling him was that when people look at me, I want them to see me for me and not think of anything bad associated with me. My academic and professional achievements must outweigh the sexual abuse of my childhood and this is the simplest reason why: because I am more than what was done to me. The only other person who knows about my past, other than my counsellor and husband, is my acupuncturist – I thought it would help me if she knew and it has helped tailor my acupuncture sessions. No one else knows about the abuse. Thankfully, with the support from my counsellor and a dedicated gynaecologist, I can now move forward.

After my two year 'break', I felt some of my pains returning, so my gynaecologist put me on Zoladex® injections. I was given the injections for six months. In that time, I was starting to feel like my well-being tank was filling back up, enough for me to return to IVF. I found a new private clinic and then the pandemic happened.

When the first UK lockdown ended, I decided to collect my three frozen embryos from the South Coast and bring them to my new clinic in London. I was so happy I had these three beauties. I collected them myself. I secured the dry shipper containing the embryos in my car and spoke to them driving up to London. I was in the process of preparing myself for a transfer with my OBGYN. Unfortunately, my three embryos did not survive the thawing process. I was devasted – my security blanket was gone. This was a huge lesson to me. Speaking to my counsellor, she said something that made sense: that I was a different person when I made those embryos and the person I am today is someone wiser and more self-aware.

I moved forward, preparing for egg collection, and during the scans they often mentioned that I had fibroids and I thought 'oh no, my old friends are back'. I asked my clinic for my scan photos and I showed them to my gynaecologist, who said that what they're seeing is, in fact, an adenomyoma, which looks like a fibroid. Thankfully, since my laparoscopy in 2017, my multiple, problematic fibroids have not returned. I don't have a definitive answer as to why this is the case, but I think focusing on myself during my two-year break helped lessen any stress and worries I had. I no longer experience the feeling of knots tightening in my belly.

So, a bit more detail about my conditions: adenomyosis and adenomyoma.

Adenomyosis affects the inner lining of the uterus (the endometrium) which breaks into the muscle wall of the uterus (the myometrium). Currently, adenomyosis is a condition that is not very well understood. There are some likely causes; however physicians cannot give a definitive answer on what causes it or the best way to treat it. Focal adenomyosis is a type of adenomyosis which occurs in one area of the uterus. Diffuse adenomyosis (what I have) is adenomyosis which has spread around the uterus. It's different to endometriosis in that operating on adenomyosis is not something that is routinely advised, as there is a risk of damaging the womb.

An adenomyoma is often mistaken for a fibroid; it is a considerable region of adenomyosis which results in a benign tumour.

In some women, adenomyosis can cause mild symptoms to no symptoms. Some of my symptoms have included: heavy bleeding, frequent urination, bulky uterus, bowel pain, severe pelvic pain, and infertility.

In terms of treatment, a common option for someone with adenomyosis is a hysterectomy. Other treatments include painkillers and anti-inflammatory drugs. It's a good idea to speak to your doctor about what pain medication would be best for you. As I mentioned earlier, hormone treatments similar to Zoladex® help to give some relief. Home treatments such as rest, heat pads, improving dietary choices, pelvic massages, pelvic exercises, and turmeric and ginger tea help. Castor oil packs (not during your period) and if you can, low impact exercises such as taking short walks. Deep breathing meditations whilst placing my warm hands on my uterus is really comforting. I love beautiful smells and I have my favourite essential oils that are calming. The pain with adenomyosis is debilitating, however it's nice to have coping mechanisms in place for those difficult days.

Every stimulation cycle I go through leaves me quite ill. The drugs used to grow the follicles for egg collections can aggravate adenomyosis. I had no idea about this when I started IVF in 2016. After egg collections, I am often left with a bulkier, painful uterus. I now take breaks between cycles to allow some time for any pain to settle.

One complication I've had since re-starting my IVF journey, is that for the past year, my right ovary has been hiding behind my uterus, which means my fertility clinic struggle to access some of the follicles. Scans have been extremely painful on the right side. I asked a few people in my fertility clinic whether the ovary could be moved, and they said no, absolutely not.

I decided to get a 'sixth opinion' on this and contacted my consultant gynaecologist. Two weeks after my conversation with him, I was booked in for a laparoscopy and he was able to successfully move my ovary from behind my uterus. Carefully cutting away any adhesions, he was able to move the ovary to a more accessible position and secured it in place. Adhesions are a type of scar tissue the body produces as it heals from trauma, such as previous surgery or infections. Adhesions can cause different organs and tissues to stick together. In some people, adhesions cause no issues but, in my case, I was experiencing pain. I can only imagine what skill it would have taken to move this ovary so I feel incredibly lucky. Four weeks post-surgery, my consultant carried out a transvaginal scan and there was my right ovary in all her glory!

This is where I am now on my TTC journey, at 38 years old. I have two more egg collections planned for the coming months and based on the evidence, the current advice for women with adenomyosis is to have single, frozen embryo transfers, with three months of Zoladex® before any transfers. Which protocol is best for you can be discussed with your fertility clinic. It's well documented that women with adenomyosis are at higher risk of miscarriage. I have thought about this and have consciously built a supportive, multi-disciplinary team to help me through my whole journey. I have found people who understand how to manage adenomyosis should I fall pregnant.

I genuinely believe, no matter what happens moving forward, that my faith in doctors has been restored. I have what I call my 'A-Team' of trusted people. I am being treated with dignity and respect. When my frozen embryos did not survive the thawing process, the first thing my consultant gynaecologist said to me was, 'I am sorry'. During a recent scan at my fertility clinic, a clinician said to me: 'I am sorry for all you have suffered'. From a young child, I simply thought pain was normal. When clinicians look inside me during surgery or when I have transvaginal scans, it is clear that my body has been hurt and damaged over the years, and it makes me sad that others can see the damage. I often think, 'What assumptions are my doctors making about me?'. Although, I fully understand that my gynaecologist and fertility clinic don't have the time to consider those things. However, being infertile has often made me question if I did something wrong at some point.

I was emotional when I saw the photos from my recent laparoscopy. I could not stop looking at the pictures and I had to remind myself that I was looking inside my body. I realised how disconnected from our bodies we can become. Many women with gynaecological pains can end up feeling anger towards their womb and I have always felt that this is an area of ourselves we need to learn to love. During the lock down, I connected with my body during walks, thanking it for carrying me and helping me to survive. Seeing the photos helped me to see what my clinicians see and to have more compassion for myself.

Forgiveness for everything that has happened in my life – many assume that must have been the most difficult thing I've had to do. I believe that I crossed the threshold of forgiveness long before I started counselling in 2018. I had some things that upset me, like many people experience, but I did not have anything in my heart to be truly angry about. I had things to work on personally and I did. I was called a 'fibroid making machine' by a gynaecologist once – I believed this about myself for years, but in fact it hasn't proven to be the case. Despite the adenomyosis, the fact that I do not make these huge fibroids anymore shows how much I have let go of. I have learned huge lessons from my past. The peace I have acquired in recent years has allowed me to tune into my intuition, that feeling in your gut that just tells you if something is right or wrong. I always had it, but I learned to ignore it. I do not ignore my intuition anymore. It's important to set energetic boundaries if you're in anyway sensitive (as I am); practice protecting yourself. I mention this because I wish I knew how to protect myself throughout my life, it's something anyone can learn to do. What keeps me on an even keel right now on my TTC journey is that I have an outstanding support network in my home life, counsellor, acupuncturist, GP who oversees my pain management, OBGYN specialising in miscarriages and last but not least, a consultant gynaecologist who is making the impossible possible.

Whilst writing this, I was thinking about my whole gynaecological health journey and reflected upon the fact that if I removed my current gynaecologist from the equation, it would be like pulling the thread on a blanket and the whole thing would fall apart. I needed a gynaecologist who was going to listen, not just see black and white but also consider the colours in between. It is super difficult to find doctors that dedicated, and I take nothing for granted. Whatever happens for me from here, I am eternally grateful to him for giving me the space to be vulnerable, without feeling frightened or nervous about any kind of discrimination or judgement. The NHS are amazing but with my plans of going through IVF again, having adenomyosis and getting a bit older, going private was the option I knew would give me some flexibility. I needed a more tailored approach to IVF. To find a gynaecologist I could sit with, I worked seven days a week in pain and made time to do the research. I can say, hand on heart, that I can breathe knowing I am in good hands. I guess my point is that I made a lot happen on this journey too, nothing was just handed to me. It is really difficult to express how it's felt for me finding my consultant gynaecologist and my best explanation is the heavens placing an angel in my path, because it's like someone up there knew I'd had enough.

I have chosen to tell you my story from my perspective only. Very often, I have thought that my husband deserves better than someone who is not able to have children naturally. I have even asked him, with clarity, if he would like to leave me and find someone to have children with, because the problem is with me. What I can say about my husband is that he wants nothing more than for me to be happy. We give each other room to grow, learn and to become the best people we can be. He did not take me up on my offer of leaving me! My husband is mentally strong, he really is, and has tackled this IVF journey head on, like a rugby scrum pushing towards that try line.

My husband decided to sponsor the education of a little boy from China some years ago and they write to each other. This little boy has now grown into an amazing teenager and I thought about the difference my husband made in this boy's life. The relationship he built with his sponsored child inspired me. I felt that I might be able to tap into motherhood through sponsoring children. I currently sponsor the education of two amazing children in Africa and we have such a great relationship. We have kept in touch throughout the pandemic and I can see their progress. They draw me pictures and I make sure they have everything they need for school. If we weren't in a pandemic, I would have liked to visit them. Perhaps this is my way of telling myself that no matter what happens in the TTC journey, there are many ways to share the love that I have. It's been an amazing experience getting to know my two angels in Africa and to buy them gifts and things for school, and I cannot wait to watch them grow up. They are already a huge part of my life. I believe education is a gift that no one can take from you. One day, I would like to sponsor more children around the world.

What happened to me as a child, and as a patient in my early twenties trying to get help, has helped me reach out more in my everyday life and in my job as a clinician. I provide my patients of all ages and backgrounds with a level of care that everyone should have access to. I would never want anyone to feel as lost as I did, and for as long as I did. In the TTC community, I have been there when people have received devastating news and reaching out is the first thing I know how to do. We send each other gifts and flowers, we exercise together, we organise baby showers and sadly, we also support women through the funerals of their babies. It is a really important community. I can honestly say that I've made life-long friends. I have days where I think, 'I am not good enough or worthy' and then there are days where I make a difference in someone's life and I think to myself, 'I have exactly everything it takes to be the best mum'. I am guilty of being self-critical, so one day I did an exercise where I wrote down positive words about myself and when I read over the words, I am reminded of who I am. I look at those words whenever I doubt my worth. I am a natural explorer; I love finding hidden waterfalls around the UK. I love exercising and really good food. Though my natural ability to have children was taken away from me, my dreams and happiness, and my constant need to be and do better, were never stolen from me.

IVF can take a toll on some relationships and can put a strain on everything, especially in a situation like mine, where it feels like I have been trying to get answers for many years. My husband and I make time for each other away from appointments and injections, and that matters. I have been on this journey since I knew something didn't feel right over 15 years ago. We will be married 10 years soon and for a young marriage, we have faced many mountains together. I have not shared my journey with my family and I am happy with that decision. My husband has told his family a little bit about what is going on.

As I write this, I do not have an ending for you. I hope I fall pregnant soon and if I do, I will share that. If it does not work for me, I will have no regrets. Beyond TTC, my amazing A-Team helped me to learn, grow and to believe in something bigger. I have a time limit in mind for how long I will pursue TTC, as adenomyosis is an incredibly painful condition to live with. Eventually, myself and my husband might need to step back and consider a future potentially without children. I have asked myself more recently: 'What would a life without children look like for me?'. It has been important for my own sanity to have a rough cut-off point but for now, the journey continues, my story continues. What the future holds is a surprise and I, for one, am excited about the next chapters.

Remember, you are not alone. No matter what your story is, there's someone else out there with the same fears and worries as you. Do not be afraid to reach out. Get support, build a support team, include pets in your support team – some women have bought a soft cuddly toy to bring with them on their journey. You create your support team. Finally, and most importantly, have faith and have hope, not just in your journey but in yourself.

Reach out to me on Instagram: @knowingmemarie

My DMs are always open.

Chosen charity

My charity is The Survivors Trust:
www.thesurvivorstrust.org/pbpaftercsa

Sexual abuse is something that no one should have to deal with alone. The Survivors Trust is a charity that helps to support survivors of sexual abuse. I have chosen this charity because the work they do is incredible. Part of their work is preparing women who have experienced childhood sexual abuse for pregnancy, birth and parenthood. Every expectant mother who has suffered in their childhood should have access to these online resources and to this wonderful charity.

Jocelyn

Jocelyn is a solo-mum-by-choice to her baby boy, born in the summer of 2020. She shares her experiences of premature ovarian failure, egg freezing, and trying for a baby using donor sperm and eventually, donor eggs as well.

Jocelyn

I'm Jocelyn, I'm 41 as I write this, and I've lived in London for the past twentyish years, working in various marketing and management roles for digital agencies. I'm mum to a little boy who's eight months old.

I found out the hard way that making a baby can be much more challenging than my schoolteachers led me to believe. When you're single and have no one to make a baby with, it's even trickier. And when you find you're almost infertile as well, it can seem impossible.

If you'd told me ten years ago that I'd be a solo mum, I wouldn't have believed you. I'd figured, like most women I know, that meeting someone, getting married, and having a couple of babies, would just naturally happen over time. I remember idly planning it out with my best friend one day when we'd just left Uni – we'd be engaged by our mid-twenties, married by 28, baby by 30 (30! Inconceivably ancient!). It all seemed so straightforward. And all through my teens and twenties I was in relationships, with one long-term boyfriend after the other. But never 'the one'. Or at least never the one I felt ready to commit to, and as I hit my early thirties, I found myself on my own for the first time. So much for the plan.

I knew that I wanted children though. It wasn't a clock-ticking, feeling broody thing, just a constant certainty that I'd be a mum one day. I've always loved kids: at weddings I'd be the one on the dance floor twirling little girls around, the first to hold the baby brought into the office. The proud godmother. So, in 2012, when I was 33, I started looking into egg freezing – just as a back-up, an insurance policy, a sensible plan B. I knew absolutely nothing about the process. It was just something I'd heard about, mostly through the media. A very modern solution to fertility preservation. A search on Google led me to the HFEA website, and I shortlisted a couple of clinics and contacted one to find out more. I wasn't in any hurry though (although, with hindsight, I blimmin' well should have been) and before I got round to actually doing anything, life took a turn, and the chance came up to go and work in America.

At the end of 2014, I was back in London for a visit and booked in to have an initial consultation at the clinic I'd found. Things got off to a bad start when the consultant's first words were: 'So, you're here to have a baby' (no, I'm here because I've nobody to have a baby with). I'd been sent a load of info, which I'd read, but this world of fertility treatment was brand new to me and the terminology was completely baffling. The doctor was speaking a different language – the language of IVF – which I'm fluent in now, but at the time I just couldn't get my head around it. The level of assumed knowledge was so high, and I was a novice. So much so, that I hadn't realised the initial blood test and scan couldn't be done if you were on any form of contraception, as I was. Looking back, this seems blindingly obvious, but at the time I was dredging my memories of GCSE biology to remember how my menstrual cycle worked, what a follicle was, and what hormones did. I was woefully ill-equipped. As a society, we are undoubtedly failing women, and men, on this front. I knew so little about my own body. I'd been taught basic reproduction, and how NOT to have a baby, and that was about it. I came away feeling a bit embarrassed and deflated, and none the wiser about my fertility.

When I came home to London the following year, I was 36. I hadn't found a boyfriend on the streets of New York, so I was still single, and thinking more and more about the future.

I went back to the clinic and had the initial fertility tests: a blood test to check FSH and AMH levels and a scan to count antral follicles. My fertility, I assumed, would be average at worst. There were women in my family who'd had babies into their forties, and I had no health issues, so I wasn't worried at all.

I was wrong.

My test results were terrible. Using charming descriptions like 'premature ovarian failure', the doctor explained that my ovaries were running out of eggs. 'We'd expect to see these results in someone ten years older than you,' she said. I was stunned. She went on to explain that egg freezing might not actually be possible at all, because my egg quantity was so low and I might not respond to stimulation: 'If you want to have a baby naturally, you'd better get on with it in the next six months'. Not very useful advice when you're single. I was devastated. The news was such a blow. And such a shock. I'd just not considered that I might find a problem. Egg freezing was supposed to only be a back-up but instead, it might be my only chance. I might never have a child. Or at the very least, I was never going to have a child in the straightforward way that I'd always imagined.

However small the chance, I felt I had to take it, and so I went ahead with the plan to freeze eggs, kicking things off in January 2016. Weirdly, until that point, I hadn't really thought of egg freezing as being like IVF but of course the process is pretty much the same, except the eggs get frozen rather than fertilised. Knowing nothing about fertility treatment, I'd prepared for the cycle by drinking copious amounts over Christmas and buying a new flat. Booze and stress – not ideal. My palms were sweating as I prepped the first injection and jabbed my stomach with the needle. After a week or so of stimulation though, it looked like only one egg might make it, so the clinic advised abandoning the cycle, which I reluctantly did (wasting hundreds of pounds on non-returnable drugs in the process).

On the recommendation of a friend and colleague, I decided to try a different clinic, and started another cycle later in the spring. This clinic did things totally differently. No more standard instructions to go away, take the drugs, and come back in ten days. This was intense and tailored, like an IVF boot camp of early morning tests and scans and personalised protocols. Things went reasonably well – better than that first try, at least – and I had a handful of eggs collected and frozen. I was learning though, that IVF can be a bit of a numbers game. A handful of eggs wasn't going to be enough – I needed multiple cycles and multiple collections to give myself a fighting chance. So, I carried on, and later that year did another egg freezing round to collect a few more.

As I learned more and more about (in)fertility that year (and got more and more desperate), I threw myself into trying to optimise the quality of the few eggs I had left: I cut down on alcohol, sugar and gluten, took various vitamins and supplements, had acupuncture once a week. I went for specialist massage to promote abdominal blood flow and practiced it at home too. I even switched my cosmetics and cleaning products to lower the chemicals I might be exposing myself to. I read books and blogs and posts, and the more I learned, the more pressure I felt to get things 'right'. So much effort, so much worry, and so much MONEY. Did any of it make any difference? I have no idea.

I'd told myself I'd probably do three rounds of freezing to try and bank a good number of eggs for potential future baby-making. So, in early 2017, I was gearing up for that third round, but I kept putting it off. My heart just wasn't in it and I couldn't put my finger on why. Just after my 38th birthday, I sat in my kitchen on a Sunday afternoon thinking about it. I ran through the familiar calculations… 'If I meet someone this year (which is unlikely because I hate dating), then maybe we'd try for a baby next year, and maybe I'd be pregnant the year after…' and so on. It was obvious I was running out of time. An idea emerged… to skip the egg freezing, and the relationship, and go straight for the baby. In the space of a few hours it went from a vague thought, to a definite plan. I couldn't remember being more excited about anything in a very long time.

Once I'd made the decision, I couldn't wait to get started. I wasn't worried about what people might think, but I was nervous about telling my parents. I feared that solo motherhood via a sperm donor might seem a bit radical, but I'd underestimated them – they were nothing but supportive. In fact, I've not encountered any negativity about my choice to go solo, although I do think the media narrative around solo motherhood, and around egg freezing, needs to change. So often, egg freezing is portrayed as a failsafe way of delaying parenthood – especially for 'busy career women'. Yet I've not come across a single woman who's embarked on solo parenthood for that reason. It's a lazy and inaccurate stereotype.

After a chat with my clinic, I set about choosing a sperm donor. Browsing profiles of potential strangers to make a baby with is a particularly surreal experience. It's like some sort of next-level dating app. I'd chosen an American sperm bank because they offered so much more information about the donors than clinics in the UK were able to. I could compare physical characteristics like height and hair colour, peruse psychological profiles, and even check out photos of donors as children and as adults. Choosing seemed impossible. I even made a spreadsheet and scored my shortlist against different criteria, but in the end, I went with the cute one with a Labrador. After a brief wrangle with my conscience about him being 23 years old (so young! Am I old enough to be HIS mother?) I made the call and paid the money.

As a stranger's sperm was flown across the Atlantic to London, I cracked on with the preparations for IVF. I had the mandatory implications counselling, which threw up some cheery points to consider, like writing a will in case I died in childbirth. And I had a round of very expensive blood tests to check various things to do with my immune system (thyroid, cytokines and natural killer cells). The general reasoning is that your immune system has to be balanced and functioning well in order for your body to successfully accept and grow an embryo. My NK cells and cytokines were both high. 'Why,' I asked my acupuncturist one day, 'is that bad? Surely a strong immune system is a good thing?'. 'Yes,' she said, 'but yours is like a lairy drunk bloke in a pub, picking fights with everyone. We need him to just sit down and chill out.'

Makes sense to me, but the whole field of

reproductive immunology is definitely contentious and although my clinic really focused on it, others ignore it completely. Getting my immunes to acceptable levels for embryo transfer would prove to be one of the most frustrating, expensive, and time-consuming parts of the whole IVF process for me, and it took a good few months before I was OK'd to start an IVF cycle in October 2017.

IVF boot camp began again, but my ageing ovaries struggled – only two eggs were collected and only one fertilised. But I still had the seven eggs, painstakingly collected and frozen from the previous rounds, to thaw and fertilise as well. The next day, the embryologist called with an update. In what was possibly the most upsetting moment of my whole infertility experience, she said: 'Oh, didn't anyone call you yesterday? None of your frozen eggs survived.'

Gutted doesn't come close to how I felt. I hadn't expected all the eggs to make it, but I definitely hadn't expected to lose all of them. All that effort, time, preparation, emotion and money. A year spent creating a chance that just completely backfired. I thought perhaps I'd had unrealistic hopes, but a few weeks later, in my follow-up appointment, I was told I'd just been really unlucky: the chance that none of my eggs survived was probably just a few percent. And there wasn't an obvious reason why the IVF hadn't worked – my immunes levels were OK, the embryo was good, everything was seemingly fine. 'You're not old,' the doctor said, 'you just have old eggs. Perhaps you'd consider using someone else's?'

I'd already talked to my sister about the possibility of her being a donor. If I couldn't make a baby from my DNA, using hers seemed the next best thing. Unfortunately, it turned out we have crap fertility in common – her test results, although a little better than mine, weren't good enough to allow her to be a donor.

By this point, it was the end of 2017. A new year was approaching and I had a plan… spend 2-3 months getting ready, and then give it one more go with my own eggs. It was time for the kitchen sink. I added DHEA and Chinese herbs to the mix, in the hope of boosting egg quality, and shipped another load of blood off to Chicago to check my immunes. The results came back high again, and a frustrating wait of several months entailed while we tried to get my cytokines down. Intralipid infusions didn't work so I was put on hydroxychloroquine (an antimalarial, weirdly) but that didn't do the trick either. My hormones were looking OK though, so in May we went ahead, with the aim of creating embryos to freeze and come back to once my immunes were better. A cocktail of Fostimon®, Merional®, Cetrotide®, Clexane®, aspirin, Viagra®, hydroxychloroquine, dexamethasone and Clomid® produced two eggs, which fertilised and went into the freezer.

I was given HUMIRA® (most often used for arthritis) and by August, something – the HUMIRA®, hydroxychloroquine, acupuncture, supplements, low stress, or possibly complete chance – brought my cytokines down to a borderline OK level. Preparations for a frozen transfer began, the two little embryos were popped back in and I kept my fingers crossed through another two-week wait. But it wasn't to be, and I tested negative again.

It's easy to sum up those eighteen months as: 'I had two cycles of IVF'. What's harder to convey is the gruelling detail of what that means. During a cycle, I'd set an alarm for 5am so I could inject myself with Cetrotide®, a drug to hold off ovulation. Then I'd get up and go to the clinic for a 7:30am blood test, to check my oestrogen and progesterone levels. I'd go to work and wait for the call to tell me what drugs to take – the dose and timing would vary each day, depending on the results of the blood test. I'd make up the injections, then give myself the jabs, wherever I happened to be at the time they said to take them: in the office, at the theatre, in Regents Park, in the Homebase car park… Every other day, I'd have a trans-vaginal scan to check the progress of the follicles. Then, in the second week of treatment, it'd ramp up to two blood tests a day, plus one or two scans. A final 'trigger shot' and then egg collection 36 hours later, under sedation. Fingers crossed for good, mature eggs, which then fertilise. An agonising wait over several days to see if the embryos develop. Then the transfer of one or two of those and another excruciating two-week wait to find out if it's worked. During which time I'd inject progesterone every night with a two-inch needle, take another two blood thinning injections and various pills, and shove about six progesterone pessaries a day up my backside. IVF is anything but glamorous. And all the while, watching what I ate, what products I used and, of course, shunning alcohol.

Going through IVF on my own was tough. I had so much support and encouragement from friends, family and my workmates too, but in the end, there was always the knowledge that quite simply, nobody else wanted it as much I did. Nobody else was as emotionally, physically or financially invested. Lots of people cared a great deal, of course, but still, it felt pretty lonely at times. Sitting in the clinic amongst the couples, I'd often be aware that as a solo mum (to be) I was in a minority (albeit a growing one). Lots of little things along the way served as reminders of that. The receptionists who called me 'Mrs'. The nurse who told me when my partner should provide his sperm sample. The doctor who suggested I go home and talk things over with my husband. Nobody meant to offend, but emotions run high through IVF (as do hormones and stress levels), and those little things did sting.

I can't know, of course, whether it would have been easier to go through IVF with a partner. It's such a demanding, exhausting, relentless process and it definitely would have been nice at times to have someone with me for all the calls and consultations, to decipher all the info and advice, to help make decisions and manage the drugs. I'm so thankful for the people close to me who did support me through those things. Being by myself has also had its upsides though. I've never had to compromise, or to consider someone else in my decisions. And I've never felt guilty for not being able to have a child, or frustrated with a partner who can't understand my point of view. I've been totally in control (well, as much as anyone can be through IVF) and I've felt fortunate in that.

By late 2018, the fact that my fertility was that of someone in their mid-late forties rather than thirties was becoming plainly evident. It was looking less and less likely that having a baby with my own eggs was going to be possible, and I'd had to rule out my sister's eggs too. The next step was to consider using an anonymous donor instead. In my head, I could hear the words of a fertility counsellor I'd seen right in the beginning, before my first egg freezing cycle. She'd asked if I'd thought about creating embryos using donor sperm and freezing those instead of eggs, as embryos tend to thaw more successfully. I'd laughed. 'Oh no,' I'd said. 'If I have a baby it'll be when I'm with a partner, so we'll use his sperm. I couldn't use a donor.' Oh, the irony.

Another new year was looming and I needed to know I had a plan in place. I signed up with an organisation that recruits altruistic UK donors and matches them to recipients. They warned me it could take time. There's a shortage of egg donors in the UK – a big reason why lots of people choose to go abroad for treatment – and it can take months. But I was lucky. I was matched with a donor in March 2019. Reading the donor's profile was a weird experience. I'd hoped there'd be an instant sense of 'she's just like me!', but there wasn't. My donor seemed very different. There were some vague physical similarities, but her background, education and career were the opposite of mine, and I had to work quite hard to remind myself that these things are superficial – they're determined to such a great extent by opportunity and circumstance, not by inherent genetic traits. I knew this woman – my donor – was kind, caring, proactive and so very generous.

When reading through donor profiles, I was often struck by how 'good' these people were. They volunteered for charity, they worked as carers, they donated blood and hair. They put me to shame! But it makes sense of course – in donating eggs and sperm they're doing one of the kindest and most generous things possible. Donors are like a self-selecting pool of lovely people. And that's a wonderful place to start when you're making a baby,

Things started to move along, and my donor was booked in for her screening tests, when another curve ball was thrown. It turned out the clinic the donor needed to be treated at couldn't accept sperm from the clinic I'd used before. So, the cute 23-year old was out. Back to the drawing board… or rather, the spreadsheet.

Choosing a sperm donor was harder this time. I tried to think of it all from the perspective of my potential, double-donor-conceived child and make choices that would be right for them. I'd used a US-based donor previously, but that no longer felt right when my egg donor was in the UK. I wanted there to be a similar level of information available about each donor, and a similar chance of my child finding them in the future, if they wanted to. But the lack of choice was frustrating and I felt much more pressure this time to get the choice 'right', because now my genes were out of the equation and I was making a baby via two (wonderful) strangers. Emotionally, it was a rollercoaster too. I still felt a bit sad about the whole thing, whilst also being excited to move forward.

I settled on a new, UK-based sperm clinic and with their help, chose a new donor. More months went by as we waited for my egg donor to be ready to begin. Finally, in October 2019, a perfect little embryo – created with the help of those two strangers and some talented doctors – was transferred to me and I waited, again. That two-week wait was a rough ride. I didn't believe the transfer had worked (and then I felt bad for not being more positive). I couldn't believe, after all I'd been through, that I'd be lucky enough to ever get a good result. I was irritable, tearful and sensitive, and I definitely didn't feel pregnant. It turned out, though, that I was. Unbelievably, amazingly, pregnant at last.

I loved being pregnant. I loved my body getting bigger and the feeling of my baby wriggling inside. Despite the rocky road I'd trodden to get to this point, I wasn't overly anxious about things that might go wrong. In a way, I figured I'd used up all the bad luck and, apart from gestational diabetes and a global pandemic interfering with my plans, I was right. When the first coronavirus lockdown came into place, I was about 22 weeks pregnant and while I hated the sudden uncertainty of how my maternity care and birth plans might be affected, I did find my experiences of going solo stood me in good stead. Suddenly everyone was having to attend scans and appointments by themselves and face the prospect of being alone in a hospital. To me, those things felt normal! When I finally found myself labouring through the night by myself (Covid restrictions meant my sister wasn't allowed on the antenatal ward with me), I knew I could draw on the strength within myself and the resilience I'd developed over those years of trying to conceive.

In July 2020, I finally met my son. My baby boy, made of magic and science and love. It sounds like a cliché, but the second he was placed on my chest, I adored him. I'd been so worried that I wouldn't feel the 'right' things, that for whatever reason I just wouldn't like my baby once he was here – that the lack of a genetic connection would mean that somehow I didn't recognise him, or warm to him, or that we wouldn't 'click'. And that fear felt horrible, especially after all the effort, time and expense it had taken to get pregnant.

People told me not to worry, but how could they know? My circumstances were so uncommon – solo mum, double donor baby – that their reassurance meant nothing. I tried to accept that the process of going down the donor route to conception is just that: a process. You don't just make the decision and never think about it again. There are lots of feelings you have along the way, and it's easy to think you should be 'over' those things (especially once you're pregnant, I found) but it doesn't work like that. It's complicated and takes time. Even once I'd committed to the donor route, there were times when I'd question my decision, or feel sad about it, right up until my son was born. It didn't mean that I'd made the wrong choice, it was just a natural part of coming to terms with taking a different path.

I needn't have worried. My son's genetic makeup hasn't made the slightest bit of difference to my experience since he was born. And I actually find the fact he's not genetically 'mine' fascinating – I can't wait to watch him develop and see what he's like. I'm so grateful for the gift my donors gave me. I hope that they know he's arrived, and I wish they could know how happy he makes me and how much I love him.

Being a new mum, and a solo mum, and a mum in a pandemic hasn't been easy. There have been moments when I've really wished for a partner to tag team with – to give me a break, to give me some reassurance, to help navigate nap schedules and weaning plans. I've envied couples decorating the nursery together, choosing prams, posing for family snaps, and sharing their baby's firsts. But actually, not as much as I thought I might. Mostly, I haven't missed having a partner much at all since being a mum. And I know that the grass isn't always greener – that just because my circumstances might have been different with a partner, doesn't mean they would be better. Having a baby can place an enormous strain on a relationship. I feel more relaxed about things now my son is here, and confident that at some point in the future, the right partner will show up too.

My boy fills my world now, and he is so, so worth everything I went through. He's amazing! As he grows, I hope I can help him understand how much I wanted him. How hard I tried for him. How miraculous it is that science and kindness brought him here to me. My body built him and birthed him. I can't imagine being a mum to anyone else.

Connect with me on Instagram: @motheringsolo

Chosen charity

My charity is the Donor Conception Network: www.dcnetwork.org

They are a supportive network of more than 2,000 mainly UK-based families with children conceived with donated sperm, eggs or embryos, those considering or undergoing donor conception procedures, and donor conceived people.

Kreena and Satty

Kreena is a mother to four children. She is a British Indian and overcame many stigmas and taboos to bring her family to life. Kreena and Satty's children are all born through surrogacy. She lost her fertility through both breast cancer and heart failure. Her daughter shares her genetics and was conceived using her own embryos. Her triplet sons were conceived using known, overseas donor conception.

Kreena

As I write this entry, I'm 41 years old, I have four wonderful children asleep in the room next door, and I feel a level of gratitude and contentment that I may not have known if I hadn't experienced the life-changing events of the past seven years.

I arrived in my 30s having led a fairly conventional life in the world of South Asians. I had been to University and was doing well in my career as an accountant. I was driven by success. My parents were immigrants, and I was acutely aware of the sacrifices they had made to educate me. I had seen their struggles, both financially and personally. Eventually, I saw their marriage fall apart and helped pick up the pieces when it came to rebuilding our lives.

I've not spoken to my father since I was 21 years old. My mother divorced him, and when she did, I felt such pride for her. She did what was right for her, not what her community expected of her. I guess she made it easier for me to break convention when my time eventually came.

I married my husband when I was 30 years old. After countless 'introductions', biodatas (marriage CVs) and Facebook stalkings of potential suitors, I finally decided to follow my heart. I married outside of my caste and outside of my religion, to a man I had known from my teenage years. A friend, a soul mate, a man who would stand by me amidst the most challenging of times.

I was 33 years old when I noticed the nipple on my left breast had become inverted. I had no idea that this was something I should worry about, but eventually, that inversion led me to a breast cancer diagnosis. A diagnosis that turned everything I knew upside down. The career I had created ground to a halt, friends and family disappeared. The image of beauty as I then knew it faded from sight. I lost myself, and wondered if I would ever find my way back.

The only living thing to have ever grown in my body was an aggressive tumour that tried to steal my life. This tumour was hormonally sensitive, and one of the most effective ways to keep it away (after chemotherapy and radiotherapy) was to force my body into a medical menopause – something that would make having children incredibly difficult.

Before I began chemotherapy, my oncologist sat me down and said: 'The treatment itself may affect your fertility. We could find that your ovaries become permanently damaged from the drugs we are about to give you'.

I had done my research; I knew this was coming and I had created a backup plan in my mind. 'Please can I have time to undergo IVF before we begin?' I asked him nervously.

'Kreena, my job here is to save your life, not to create a new life,' he replied.

My heart felt physically heavy. Children were always part of my life plan – I had never imagined a life without them, but then again, I had never imagined a life with cancer, so the script I had pre-written for the story of my life was well and truly torn to pieces.

We went on to talk about the risks of IVF, the fact that the drugs could encourage rogue cancer cells to grow and multiply further, the fact that my main tumour had been removed so an element of risk had been reduced. We spoke about what medication I could take alongside the IVF drugs to help keep the cancer risks to a minimum. I took it all on board; every single word that he said. I found myself wondering if I would even survive this disease, was this conversation simply academic? What if I died before any of these eventualities actually came to be?

In the end, I decided to go ahead with IVF. I was given two weeks (not a day more) to find a clinic, to find the money, find the strength and find the eggs that would hopefully one day make me a mother.

Going through IVF whilst waiting for cancer treatment was horrendous. Two of the toughest things a woman can have to deal with landing at the same time. My body changed in ways I never knew possible. I had lost one breast by this point, my femininity was slowly fading, and collecting my eggs – knowing I may never produce one again – was a painful reminder of everything I was losing.

Every day, as I injected myself in my stomach, I would pray that I didn't aggravate my cancer. Hope of a successful egg collection always came secondary to that. There was a huge cloud that hung over me, following me wherever I went. Our fertility team were great – they were empathetic to our situation and tried their hardest to make this one and only round of treatment a success. Each day, we were gently reminded that this treatment cost money, and that our CCG had not yet approved our request for funding… until one day, we walked in and felt the elephant in the room.

'I'm sorry Kreena, we've been told you won't be entitled to NHS funding for this treatment. You'll need to pay for it yourselves.'

I lived in a postcode that funded IVF treatment, however, because I arrived at infertility (or prevention of it) through cancer, I didn't meet the standard criteria of TTC unsuccessfully for two years or more. We were devastated – how unfair could the system be? If I waited a further two years, despite being funded, the chances of success would be very low. We made the decision to continue with IVF and self-fund if we had to. As the days passed, I contacted my CCG, I spoke to my GP and I raised an urgent appeal and IFR (individual funding request). I also hunted down my MP and shared my story with him. I used every bit of my energy to have the decision overturned, and as I woke on the morning of egg retrieval day, I saw an email in my inbox that made me smile for the first time in a long time. The appeal was successful – my funding was now approved and we had one less thing to worry about.

The day of our collection arrived and we were filled with fear and hope in equal measures. I would flit from a fear of dying to the hope of living every single day. From questioning if I was doing the right thing, to knowing that this had to be done to create a little insurance policy of our own. As I was taken down to theatre, my husband ran around, organising refunds onto our credit cards for the money we had already paid to the clinic. A nurse held my hand through the procedure and escorted me back to the ward when we were done. After a period of recovery, Satty and I drove home. I felt sore and uncomfortable but reminded myself that I had already endured more pain than this during my mastectomy and that everything would soon settle down.

The next day, I received a call from the embryologist: 'Kreena, we have great news: we collected 13 eggs, 12 fertilised and 11 made it to the freezer. This is excellent, you should be so proud. We wish you all the best for your upcoming treatment, do stay in touch.'

I didn't say much other than 'hello' and 'ok'. I had woken up with the 'I'm going to die' mindset and couldn't share the excitement of this lovely lady on the other end of the phone. I hung up and cried. I looked out of my bedroom window and asked myself if I had just created a life that I would never live to see.

I didn't think about those embryos that much for the months that followed. I had stepped aboard the cancer train and all of my focus and energy had to be channelled towards getting to the end of the line, the end of treatment, the end of this living nightmare. I mourned so much of myself as I navigated oncology treatment. My single, lone breast and absent hair a constant reminder of all that was gone. The good health I had taken for granted, the youthful, radiant body that was now a distant memory, the fertility I was born with that I never truly knew the value of.

I turned 35 in October 2015. I had completed my active treatment and the light at the end of the tunnel was beginning to appear. I began to look to the future. I'd been speaking to my oncologist and was reminded again and again of the risks of attempting to fall pregnant. I was on a ten-year treatment plan to avoid a cancer recurrence and a baby would require a pause in that treatment – a pause that my team advised would be too high risk. I had been researching alternate routes to motherhood; every time, I came back to surrogacy. I was both intrigued and fearful. How did it work? How would I find someone? How would I get my family on board? Where could I find someone like me – an Indian girl who knew, understood and felt the same anxieties I did?

I never found the latter, but eventually I found the answers to all of the other questions. I'd found online forums that supported me through cancer, and those same forums introduced me to surrogacy. I spent years gathering knowledge of how surrogacy worked in the UK. I looked into agencies and attended conferences. My husband was unsure. We had no experience of this new world I had immersed myself into. There were no guarantees; it felt like there was so much risk, and on top of that, we were Indian, and Indians seemed to just procreate. It seemed effortless for all our peers – no one spoke of struggles, no one shared stories of IVF. We felt so alone, so unlucky.

I felt like I had let the side down; the issues and road blocks to a family all sat with me. The damaged goods in the marriage; the one who could probably be replaced and upgraded with a new, fully working model in the blink of an eye. I think that fear was my driver, that's what created this fire in my belly, a determination to find a way forward. By nature, I don't take no for an answer – if I want something, I will do everything in my power to get it. So, whilst my husband took his time to digest the thought of surrogacy, I armed myself with every bit of knowledge I would need for the day he found a way forward with it.

It was summer 2016 when our first surrogacy journey came to life. After being on independent Facebook forums for quite a while and meeting a number of potential surrogates (none of which worked out), I received a message from a lady called Ina. I remember her message: 'Hi, I'm Ina, I've been following you online and wondered if you were interested in getting to know one another?'

Ina's message arrived on my phone amidst some of the darkest days of my life. Having come through cancer, Satty and I had flown to Vancouver. We had planned a special holiday, a trip to celebrate the end of oncology treatment. I had two, newly built breasts, my head was full of hair once again, and life was more normal than it had been in a very long time.

As we settled into the first day of our trip, I mentioned to Satty that I felt a little unwell – that my chest felt tight and I wondered if I'd picked up a bug from the flight. I took some paracetamol as we continued with our trip and spent time away with some old friends. I woke the next morning feeling more poorly, breathing felt laboured and I lacked my usual energy and enthusiasm. My chest was still tight, I had started to cough, and nausea also crept in. Twenty-four hours later, I found myself at a walk-in medical centre. I was gasping and struggling to breathe – my lungs felt like they weren't working, it felt like I was drowning.

I sat on the doctor's bed as he examined me, and before I knew what was going on, I burst into tears. 'I think I have lung cancer,' I said to him. He looked at me with confusion. He calmed me down and told me that it was highly unlikely that this was cancer, but that he was concerned. He referred me to a local hospital and requested a series of further tests.

I had an MRI and CT scan. Initially, they thought I was suffering with pneumonia, but when that was eliminated, they looked further – potentially a clot on my lungs, or something more serious. By this point, I was unable to stand and confined to a hospital bed. Eventually, I was transferred to a larger hospital – more tests, more questions. I was now slipping in and out of consciousness and had been given equipment to help me breathe, as I was unable to do this myself. Every vein in my hands and feet were pierced with needles and cannulas. Doctors came and went; nurses did all they could to keep me comfortable.

A team of medics came to the bedside and told my husband they couldn't find the cause of my illness, but that they were gravely concerned. That if this continued, he should prepare himself for the worst. He should call over any family members who may want to say their final goodbyes, because my life was hanging on by a thread and they couldn't find a way to support me or bring me back.

The very last team to come to my bedside were cardiologists. They connected me to an ultrasound machine and told me they wanted to look at my heart. I remember seeing Satty in the corner, crying; he held my left hand. Another doctor came to my right hand and held it tightly: 'Kreena, I know you are afraid and that you can barely speak, but if you can hear me, and understand me, please squeeze my hand.'

I heard him but didn't see him. My eyes were too heavy to open.

'Can you remember if the chemotherapy you were given three years ago was red in colour? If it was, please squeeze my hand.'

My mind shot back to the chemo ward, to my nurse next to me, a syringe of red liquid in her hand that carried a huge toxicity label. I had asked her why she sat with me for the whole infusion. She told me that this drug, Epirubicin, was particularly harsh. That it had a number of serious side effects she needed to look out for, but that it was also hugely effective in treating my type of cancer. I'd sat back and watched the red liquid disappear from the syringe into my body, no thought or concern for any of those side effects, because at that moment, my priority was its effectiveness at treating my cancer.

I squeezed the hand of the cardiologist by my bedside. At the same time, the entire team gravitated towards the ultrasound machine. Within seconds, a button was pressed, and a siren went off above my head. Tears streamed and streamed from my eyes, Satty's grip on my hand became tighter.

'She is in acute heart failure, get her to Cardiac ICU immediately.' The barriers around my bed were lifted, the brakes unlocked, and like something out of the movies, I was whisked away.

Heart failure – what did that even mean? Would I die in the next few hours? The next few days? How did anyone survive with a failed heart? Would I need a transplant to live? How would I possibly find a match in time? How was this happening? How was I facing death again for the second time in three years? What about this man next to me, what would happen to him?

I made it through that night. The following morning, I woke up. I felt better than the day before. A doctor came to my room and told me she was a cardio-oncologist. I had no idea what that meant, but she told me she specialised in cancer and heart disease. She told me that she believed chemotherapy had damaged my heart, and there was no magic remedy to fix it immediately. My heart function had dropped to 6%, the muscle itself was hugely dilated. It was becoming impossible to pump blood around my body, and fluid had built up in my lungs.

'We're not quite sure how you are still here, or how you're even coherent. You are one strong woman and we're going to do everything we can to treat you. But you need to know, the chances of surviving an incident this severe are very low.'

That evening, my sister arrived in Vancouver – she had booked a flight as soon as she'd heard the news. Her arrival to my bedside in Cardiac Intensive Care made me feel safe and afraid at the same time – safe in her arms, but afraid this would be our final goodbye.

That night, I recorded voice notes and sent messages to everyone I held close. I told them how much they meant to me, apologised for not saying goodbye in person, and made peace with the fact that this could be where my story ended.

I survived the critical period of my life in Cardiac Intensive Care, I made it out of the unit and onto the ward, and from there, I was eventually discharged. A restricted diet, no salt consumption, limited water to be drunk, and a wheelchair for my mode of transport. It certainly wasn't the dream holiday we had planned, but it was a chance to live, and one I chose to grab with both hands.

It took almost two months for my body, and the medical team, to allow me to fly home to the UK. I boarded the flight with an oxygen tank to hand, a nurse by my side, and a fear that ran through me. My heart had to hold out; I had to get home. I wanted to see my mum, I wanted to see my loved ones. As we touched down at Heathrow airport, I breathed a huge sigh of relief – finally, we were home.

The next nine months were a very slow but very steady transition back to some sort of normality. I was under the care of an incredible cardio-oncologist in London and together, we worked relentlessly to get my heart pumping again and to get me back on my feet.

It was during those days in Vancouver where my relationship with Ina began. She continued to talk to me, she gave me hope. A total stranger, who wasn't really interested in how unwell I was, she simply wanted me to find a way to enjoy the country we found ourselves stranded in. That was hugely uplifting.

My return to the UK and cardiac rehab brought with it the next chapter of our lives. Ina and I had continued to stay in touch; we met individually and then with our families. We both became more engrossed in the Facebook communities we were now a part of. Both researching, both equipping ourselves with the knowledge we would need if we were to match.

In the UK, surrogacy is regulated, but there are no surrogacy specific laws in place. Arrangements cannot be commercial in nature and a surrogate is only allowed to claim expenses from her Intended Parents. It can be carried out independently or via an agency. Anyone entering a surrogacy arrangement is advised to do so with an agreement in place. The agreement details the expectations that each party has of one another. From practical things, such as when expenses payments need to be made, to the tragedy of how to deal with miscarriage or still birth. Whilst the agreement isn't legally binding, the parties create it from a place of trust and it forms the basis of any surrogacy journey.

Ina and I were both first-timers, so there was a lot to get our heads around. The existing laws, how parental responsibility is treated after the child is born, how much we wanted to see each other, how involved we all wanted to be.

The embryos we had harvested ahead of chemotherapy were stored at a clinic in London. The clinic didn't hold a surrogacy licence, so we found a clinic that would work for us as a team and had them transferred. I remember the day of transfer so clearly. The embryos that I once rejected, the ones that once filled me with fear, now held all my hopes and dreams. I was petrified that something would go wrong. That our courier would be involved in a road traffic accident, that something would take those maybe babies and my last shot at motherhood (as I perceived it to be back then) away from me.

Fortunately, the embryos arrived safely at our new clinic. Ina, myself and my husband met with our team to lay out our plans for TTC. We were each given separate consultations to ensure that we were on the same page. We were referred to a counsellor, who went on to independently assess us, ensuring that no one was being forced into the arrangement and that everyone understood the process and the risks.

After that, we found ourselves on the treatment train, but there didn't seem to be a specific station for surrogacy. We signed endless reams of paperwork, all of which seemed to repeat itself, or refer to donor conception. There was little or no mention of forms specifically drafted for a surrogacy arrangement.

We were given a list of blood tests that needed to be carried out, but when we questioned their relevance, no one was able to answer our questions. For example, our embryos were created in 2013, and at that time my husband and I had both been tested for HIV. Yet ahead of treatment, we were both asked to take that test, and many others, again – despite the embryo not transferring into me, not being newly created and not changing since they were frozen in time.

I often feel like the word 'infertility' attracts a price tag. Once someone knows how desperate you are to have a baby, there's a perception that you have, or will find, any amount of money needed to make it happen. Layer surrogacy on top of that and the chargeable items never seem to end. We went with protocol, we had no other choice. Fortunately, our GP was great and carried out a number of tests on the NHS. Those that couldn't be done with her, were paid for privately at the clinic.

We had planned a medicated cycle with Ina. We knew that we had a finite number of embryos, that there was no option to collect more eggs and that we needed to give the transfer every bit of help we could. As an Intended Parent, that's an easy decision to make, you want to do anything you can to improve the chances, but when the person having to take those drugs is not you, you have to ensure that they're on board.

Ina struggled with the IVF drugs – as a healthy woman who knew she could conceive and carry a pregnancy, I know there were times when she wished the medication could be stopped. But we all knew it served a purpose; we knew we wanted this to work. Ina was incredible, and I was in awe of what she was willing to put her body through to make me a mother.

Our first round of treatment didn't work. Ina's lining wasn't thick enough so we took a break and tried again a few weeks later, with more hormones added to the mix. This time, everything looked better. Ina was attending a clinic that was local to her for blood tests and scans, then feeding the information back down to the clinic we were being treated at. There were 200 miles between us and an awful lot of red tape to get through. I became chief of admin: meticulously counting days, searching for information, chasing blood test results, ensuring everything was going to plan, that nothing was being forgotten or missed off. It was all I could do; it was all I felt useful for.

On the day of the transfer, I met Ina at the clinic. She came with her partner and her son and I went along to meet them. We encouraged Ollie to drink as much hot chocolate as he could, jesting that this would hopefully be one of our final visits here and that we needed to somehow get our money's worth from the place!

We had been tracking the progress of our embryos for the five days leading up to this point. We had paid for video monitoring and I had called the lab every morning to check in on them. We arrived on day 5 and I was taken to a side room, where an embryologist advised me that there were four or five viable embryos. One was a particularly good, day 5 blastocyst and that would be the embryo they chose for transfer.

I then went to see the consultant. We discussed the quality of the embryo and our transfer plans. He advised that we were in a good position, that we had a number of options, but that this one embryo was better than the rest and that we would proceed with transferring it into Ina. A nurse then came to Ina and called her through to theatre. She then came to ask if I wanted to join… I hesitated, and then said no. Of all the things Ina and I had discussed, we'd never discussed whether she would want me with her on transfer day. I regretted saying no the moment the nurse turned her back and walked away.

I spent the next 45 minutes wearing the waiting room floor thin, pacing up and down, counting the minutes, praying that everything was ok. Eventually, Ina walked through the doors towards us. I asked her how it went, how she was feeling? She told me that she wished I had been with her – how amazing it was to watch, to see the tiny embryo on screen before it was transferred into her. We laughed at how we had both been too shy, and how that needed to change for the rest of the journey. We stopped for some lunch and then headed our separate ways, each full of hope.

Satty and I had planned to take time out over the first weekend of our two-week wait. We knew it would be torturous and wanted to find a distraction. We jumped on the Eurostar and spent a few nights visiting Brussels and Bruges.

We waited for the clinic to call us the following morning – our remaining embryos were due to be refrozen after our transfer, but the call never came. I called again and again in the days that followed, and eventually, four days after our transfer, the phone was connected to the embryology department. I asked for an update on how the refreeze went – how many back-up options we had if this transfer failed?

'I'm sorry, Mrs Dhiman, your embryos have all perished.'

Nausea built-up inside me immediately, my heart ached and I fell to the ground. I hung up the phone and I cried a river of tears. We'd started this process with 11 embryos, now all we had left was the single one transferred into Ina. It wasn't, and still isn't, clear what happened to those embryos. When I left the clinic on day 5, there were at least four that should have made it back into the freezer. As I walked out of my consultation with the embryologist, we'd discussed refreezing later that day, yet for some reason, without our consent, they were left another day and then a decision made not to refreeze them.

That day still haunts me. Why did someone else have the right to decide what happened to my embryos? My maybe babies; my last shot at motherhood?

I called Ina as soon as I could compose myself, as she had been asking daily about our remaining embryos: 'They've gone, Ina. We have nothing left!'.

I explained the conversations and everything that happened. We were angry, we were frustrated, we cried together. I can only imagine the amount of pressure this put on Ina – her desire and need to make this last piece of hope stick and grow inside her, to still find a way to make me a mum.

Before our transfer, Ina and I had discussed home pregnancy tests at length, and we'd agreed not to do them, not to get our hopes up, just to wait for our pregnancy bloods at the clinic to confirm if our transfer was successful. Within a few days, Ina messaged me – it was a photo of pregnancy tests stacked on the supermarket shelf. We laughed and joked, we said no, we agreed no! But within a couple of days, there were pee sticks on order, and we knew we would cave!

Ina said she felt pregnant, and the day her period was due to arrive… it didn't! I allowed myself to dream; I began to wonder if we were lucky enough for our one and only transfer to work. Satty remained grounded, he told me not to tell him if Ina took a test – I was bursting. One by one, the images and videos started to ping on my phone. First, small sticks showing what looked like a positive, then one day, as I stood in a DIY store waiting to pay for a screwdriver, an image of a home test with two very clear lines on it pinged on my phone. I opened it and screeched – Satty just gave me 'The Look'. He still wouldn't look at my screen but we both knew that this could be it. Then a couple of days later, I was at hospital with my mum (who we were planning on surprising at a later stage), when another video landed.

This time, it was a Clearblue® test. Ina had recorded it from start to finish and after a minute, the word 'PREGNANT' flashed on the screen. I was so excited I could've been sick! I had never seen a pregnancy test like this one or known what to expect or see. Next came the words '2-3 weeks'. My heart was racing… I wrote back to Ina, but all I could manage was 'omg, omg, omg'… a hundred times over. My poor mum was still clueless as to why I was wearing such a big grin. It was when that test came through that I allowed myself to believe we were actually pregnant, that finally things were going our way! That this dream could finally be coming true!

We went on to have pregnancy bloods carried out, and the news was confirmed: we were indeed pregnant. Six weeks later, we arrived at the clinic for an early scan. Again, I had no idea what to expect. I went along with my amazing surrogate to see what magic we had made. We saw a sac, and the doctor pointed out that everything looked well. Ina then asked if we would see a heartbeat… then it appeared, a flashing light on the screen, nestled between the grainy black and white image. THERE IT WAS – the beginnings of our little miracle, the heart that would grow inside Ina and live on in my child. Tears filled my eyes, gratitude flowed, we hugged and held each other. Neither of us had ever seen a pregnancy scan like that, we were both blown away.

Ina and I kept in close contact through her pregnancy. We would text and send pictures to each other every week, we met up in person as often as we could. It's strange when someone else is carrying your baby – you want to be there for everything, you want to do whatever you would do if you were able to carry yourself, but you have to be mindful that this other person has a life and a family of their own too. That carrying your child takes enough of them and their energy, and that your desires as an Intended Mother simply have to take a back seat, control has to be lost for the relationship to flourish.

Ina was incredible. She kept me up to date with everything that she was going through and all of the developments with Amaala. We attended her scans and booked some private scans too. Seeing our miracle baby on screen, perfectly formed – ten little fingers, ten little toes, a perfect button nose – took my breath away.

We kept our pregnancy a secret from our friends and family. I had come up with a plan to surprise everyone once the baby was born – I'd seen some great examples on social media and decided to create them for ourselves too. In December 2017, we did however, share the news with our immediate family. On Christmas morning, I wrapped up canvas images of our baby scan and handed them to my mum and sister. They opened and looked at them in confusion – they didn't even know that we had found a match in Ina, let alone fallen pregnant. As the penny dropped, the floodgates opened – a level of joy I hadn't seen or ever experienced. The first grandchild in our family. After years – no, decades – of hurt and pain.

Being able to share that news with my loved ones was priceless, a moment I'll never forget. They had known how hard I was working to make it happen, the obstacles that stood in our way, the complexities that needed to be overcome, but here we were; we'd made it!

The questions rolled in: How did I meet Ina? When did we fall pregnant? When would the baby come home to us? How did the arrangement work? The relationship, the financials... all of it. I explained how surrogacy in the UK was altruistic, how we paid Ina pregnancy expenses each month, in ten equal installments. How the baby wouldn't legally be mine once born, but that it would be once we went through an assessment by Cafcass (Children and Family Court Advisory and Support Service) and the family courts. I told them how I trusted Ina infinitely, how our relationship was honest and strong, and that I had no fear at all of her wanting to keep the baby! In fact, she was more worried about being left holding the baby if Satty and I ever changed our minds. It was a lot of information for Christmas Day, but it was certainly one that none of us will ever forget.

In April 2018, we loaded our car and drove up the M4 for the final time as a family of two. We had rented a cottage close to Ina, in a bid to be with her when the time came for our baby to enter the world. We enjoyed our last few days of the pregnancy with Ina and her family and attended her final midwife appointment with her the week of her due date. It was there that we were told that Ina's bump had decreased in size and that the baby was dry. We were referred to the Royal United Hospital, all of us anxious and fearful. Ina and the baby were monitored, heart traces were being routinely run and we were told that Ina needed to be induced. We were only five days away from our due date and an induction seemed the safest option. We breathed a sigh of relief – we had a solution and a way to keep Ina and the baby safe.

But then the doctor turned to us and told us that the hospital was very busy and there wasn't space to admit Ina. We were advised that the best thing we could do was go home. I felt sick – we hadn't come this far to only come this far. The years we had worked to create this life, the odds we had fought, the journey we had been on… all to be told that five days before our baby was due, she was at risk and that there was no space to do anything about it.

We were sent away, and Ina was told to call the hospital if it felt like the baby was moving less than usual. Again, the pressure fell onto her shoulders and it was up to her to call out if she thought something was wrong. We left each other that evening filled with anxiety. I told Ina that we were on standby for a call at any time, day or night, if she needed to be admitted, we would be there by her side. None of us got much sleep that night, my mind was full of distraction and I checked my phone every 30 minutes to make sure I didn't miss anything.

The following morning, Ina rang the hospital. She was unsure of Amaala's movements and wanted to be checked again. She was admitted that day and the following 48 hours were the lead up to us meeting our first born, miracle baby.

Eventually, Ina was induced and went into a long and painful labour. Some of the memories that followed are a blur and some are crystal clear. Satty and I had walked away from the labour ward for some air, and when we came back, we were met by nurses telling us that Ina had progressed very quickly. That we could be meeting our baby any time soon. We were escorted down to the delivery suite, hearts in our mouths, praying we didn't miss anything, and were told to wait in a waiting room.

We both paced up and down. A midwife came to us and told us that Ina asked that we wait outside for now (this wasn't the original plan). Fear rose inside of me; I could see it in Satty's eyes too. What was going on? What had changed… was Ina ok? Was the baby ok?

There were several people in the waiting room: parents, grandparents, people taking care of small children as their mummies and daddies welcomed their siblings into the world. I noticed a feeling of being watched, like everyone was wondering what we were doing. The midwife had spoken about our baby, but how could there be a baby when I, the mother, was stood in front of them. Part of me wanted to tell them all about how a wonderful surrogate was giving birth to our child, and part of me just wanted to shut out everyone and everything around us, to only focus on Ina, our baby and both of them getting through this safely.

After a couple of hours waiting outside, we were finally reunited with Ina in her delivery room. Her pain was under control and we exchanged stories with each other. I held her hand and sat next to her, watching the monitor by her side, which was tracing Amaala's heart rate. It was slightly elevated, but not a huge cause for concern at this point.

The guys headed off to get a coffee – the labour had slowed down, and it felt like we all had a little time to breathe. Ina was telling me that, despite having an epidural, she could still feel pain in the lower left corner of her tummy and I asked the midwife what could be done to help her. Eventually, we found out that Ina's epidural catheter had come away and the localised pain she felt then spread and she could feel everything.

Ina's partner, Ivars, returned and stood by her side. Satty waited outside as things became intense in the delivery room. I stood back and watched Ina, this incredible human, in so much pain, and all for me, all to make me a mother.

On the monitor beside her bed, the baby's heart rate began to race, beeps kept going off and a sense of unease filled the room. The decision was made to get to theatre and prepare for a c-section to keep both Ina and Amaala safe. I remember feeling quite useless at the time – of no help to my wonderful surrogate, nor to my unborn child, an outsider in this room, the one person who had very little to offer.

I was afraid – afraid of something going wrong, of Ina suffering complications, of Amaala not making it. I remember thinking it was all my fault. That everyone was in this situation because of me. My inability to grow a baby. I looked at Satty as he watched from the other side of the door, wishing he was closer, wanting to spend these moments with him by my side, but knowing that my own desire came secondary to the person currently in labour.

Ina looked at me as the consent forms for the c-section were signed. We had always agreed that if we had to go to theatre, I would go with her. I watched as Ivars held her hand and comforted her. I told her that he needed to go with her, that I would wait in recovery. She said, 'But it's your baby', to which I replied, 'And this is your body, you need him.'

The midwife had caught our conversation and spoke to the consultant. 'We are allowing you both in, Ivars and Kreena. Satty, I'm so sorry you'll have to wait in recovery, but as soon as the baby is here and safe we will bring you in.'

I saw the tears fill in Satty's eyes as he agreed. Ivars and I quickly changed into scrubs and the next thing we knew, we were in theatre with Ina. The team advised me that they would be attempting delivery with forceps or a suction cup, but if those didn't work, we would be heading to a c-section. Ivars held Ina's hand. I clasped my own hands and watched Satty, as he looked in from the recovery room.

Amongst the chaos came a shift change of staff, and with it, a midwife who had cared for us for the past two days. She saw Satty alone in recovery, raised it with the consultant and 30 seconds later, he was in scrubs and sat beside me, my hand in his.

Those moments before Amaala was born felt perfect. The four of us, the team who had made this all happen, all next to each other to see the arrival of this miracle baby. We didn't need a c-section in the end.

Amaala was born with the help of some forceps, and as she entered the world, she was held in the air and I looked at Satty and cried: 'It's a girl!'. I'd spent the entire pregnancy dreaming of a daughter. Everyone around me was convinced we were having a boy, but my gut had thought it would be a girl from early on – the only name I had chosen was Amaala. And there she was, the baby I never thought would be, the one thing that had kept me going through some of my darkest days. The hope that flowed through me, the tiny little life that would go on to be my saving grace.

Satty and I took Amaala in to recovery, we held her skin to skin and breathed her in. I had always feared how I would connect with our baby once it was born. Would I immediately feel like their mother? Would they know me as their mother? What if she rejected me? Yet the moment I held her, those fears faded. I knew she was mine. I knew I would protect her, I knew that how she came to me wasn't important. What mattered now was being the best mum I could be to this little miracle baby.

That night, Ina, Satty and I stayed in the hospital. Ina had a private room and Amaala was with Satty and I on the ward. As Amaala drifted to sleep, we wheeled her over to Ina, to show her how perfectly she had grown our baby girl. Satty had packed a bottle of champagne with some plastic flutes, and we raised a glass to us, to Ina, to the magic that made this dream come true. We ordered a pizza, had our dinner together and then headed off to sleep.

Two days later, Amaala was discharged from hospital. Ina had left the day before, and Satty and I were allowed to take Amaala home without Ina having to return. We spent the next five nights in our little cottage, tucked away in the English countryside, just the three of us. Away from the excited family members waiting to meet her, away from the questions that we knew would soon flow, away from everything. Those days were quite simply, perfect.

Eventually, we made the journey home. We stopped at Ina's house to say goodbye and to let her children meet Amaala. Leaving their house that day, I was so full, so content, so proud of the journey we had been on. So grateful that it all fell into place.

Ina and her family are still a part of our lives. In the months after Amaala was born, we met to register her birth, we met again ahead of our Family Court hearing. When a child is born in the UK, the birth mother is listed as their mother on the birth certificate. In order to change that, and for Amaala to be recognised as my daughter in the eyes of the law, all parties are required to approve the application of a parental order. This meant a trip to court and an assessment by social services on my ability to parent this beautiful baby.

Ina and her family joined us for Amaala's first birthday and we've spent time together since. I speak to Amaala about Ina all the time – about how she grew in Ina's tummy and about how Ina took care of her before she came to live with Mummy and Daddy. It's important to me that she knows about her journey, the love that went into creating her, the lengths we all went to to bring her to life. I want her to understand how selfless Ina was – how without the help of a stranger, she would not be here. Because to me, it's a major life lesson. A life lesson on love and compassion, on humility and kindness, on resilience and strength. I want her to take those lessons and carry them forward into the making of the woman she will one day become.

It wasn't long after Amaala was born that we began to think of a sibling journey. I was acutely aware of how many years it had taken to bring Amaala into our lives and wanted to start having conversations to work out what we would need to do to go on another journey.

We spoke to Ina, and fortunately her thoughts had been aligned to ours. She told us that she would love to carry a sibling for us and that she would be there for us once we had worked out the finer details. We knew that we didn't have any embryos left, and therefore donor conception was going to be our only option. I took my time when it came to exploring donor eggs. It wasn't a decision that we simply woke up and decided on, there was just so much to consider.

I spent months exploring my own thoughts, understanding how I would feel having one child that was biologically mine and another who wasn't. I took time to understand that my love for Amaala didn't come from genetics, it came from the heart, from my place in her life as her mother and hers in mine as my daughter.

I briefly gave thought to a traditional surrogacy (TS) journey. In TS, the surrogate's own eggs are used and fertilised. That would have made our journey slightly simpler, but I was mindful of two things. I knew Ina was never looking for a TS journey, and at the time, having the same surrogate carry my children was a romantic notion I wasn't quite ready to give up on. I also knew that there were very few surrogates of colour in the community. A part of me wanted my next child to look as much like the rest of us as possible, so we made the decision to look for a donor.

It quickly became apparent that Indian donors are almost non-existent in the UK. That if I waited for one, we could be waiting forever. I spoke openly about our search for a donor amongst my friends within the surrogacy community, and I asked for guidance and help. So many conversations were had, so many scenarios played out in my head. One of those conversations touched on known egg donation and the use of overseas clinics and agencies to gain access to a greater pool of donors, and the ability to see a picture of a donor, maybe even meet them.

I took that information away and spent some time thinking about that route and the consequences it may have. The ability to see images of our donor would allow me to match them as closely to myself as possible, however it would remove anonymity, was I ready for that? How would that affect our future child? I was so aware that egg donation was unspoken of in the South Asian community and wondered how this might affect us and the decisions we went on to make.

I spoke to Satty and we decided to explore it further. I made contact with a clinic in Cyprus and got the ball rolling. I sent details over for what we wanted in a donor. My primary request at the time was 'someone Indian'. When our coordinator told me that they had several donors of Indian heritage available, I felt a level of excitement begin to build. At last, we had found a way forward. At last, we had the chance of making Amaala a big sister.

I read through the profiles that were sent to me and flicked through pictures. I found girls with similar features to mine, but for some reason, my gut told me they weren't the ones. I told our coordinator we would wait, that I now realised I wanted something more than just a match based on looks. The more I read profiles, the more I began to realise that this process was also about finding a connection. One day, I would meet this woman, tell her my story, show her what she was giving us, show her the family she was helping to build. I don't think I knew exactly what I wanted or needed until the right profile landed in my inbox. I guess it's like any major life event, when you know, you just know.

I remember the day I read the profile of our donor. Her opening quote told me so much about her. She was a dreamer, a believer, a hard worker. She held hope close to her heart, she believed in the universe and the role it plays in bringing people together. Her looks became secondary, I fell in love with her zest for life, her open heart that flowed from the brief bio I was sitting and reading.

Once we had committed to our donor, I became increasingly more excited. The clinic advised that only Satty needed to fly out to create our embryos, however I knew that we would travel as a family. The ability to meet this girl in person was too much to miss. The next thing we knew, we were on a plane to Cyprus. Our donor had been undergoing a medicated cycle in South Africa and had flown to Cyprus the day before us. We arranged to see her the evening of her collection and headed up to the pool to meet the person who would go on to help us complete our family.

We were planning on a ten-minute chat, an introduction to ourselves, some deep and honest thank you's and we would be on our way. That fifteen minutes turned into over two hours. Effortless conversation, a connection that words can't describe and a knowing that this was always meant to be. We took pictures together, and she asked if we would let her know if the donation resulted in a pregnancy and a baby – I told her we would be sure to keep her in the loop.

I didn't once feel intimidated by her, I didn't feel inferior because she had something I desperately needed. If we were lucky enough to have a baby, I didn't feel like keeping in touch would take away from my role as a mother. I believe that level of knowing and self-assurance was the result of our first surrogacy journey. A journey that taught me there are good people in this world; people who will give a piece of themselves to make someone else's dream come true. I had learnt to trust and surrender – two life lessons that I am grateful for.

Our donor was accompanied to Cyprus by the lady who ran the agency that introduced us. Her warmth and tenacity made our meeting memorable and easy. We all decided that one evening together wasn't enough. The following day, we met in the restaurant for breakfast and went on to spend the rest of the day together at a beachside hotel. As we parted company that day, tears were shed. We'd come to Cyprus in the hope of creating viable embryos, what we left with was beyond any of our expectations. Seven grade A frozen embryos and a relationship that would go on to last for years to come. Of course, I'm aware that not every donor story will play out in this way, that some couples will prefer a level of anonymity, but for those who do want more, there are options out there.

Our hearts were full when we arrived back home in England. It felt like everything was in place for our sibling journey to proceed. I spoke to Ina and we discussed dates for a potential transfer towards the end of the year. We celebrated life and the future we had always dreamt of.

In August 2019, I took a long overdue break with my best friend, to Juicy Mountain in Turkey, a place like no other. Our days were filled with everything that is good for the mind, body and soul. Sunrise and sunset yoga and meditation were my favourite. We would arrive at the platform, the rolling mountains lay in front of us and the sun would appear, a bright orange ball of fire. Our teacher would guide us through movement and breath work and close each session with a powerful 11-minute meditation – a meditation to manifest your dreams to life, to find your truth. Twice a day, every day, for one week, I would sit and envision my next chapter, tears would stream down my face. Silhouettes of Satty holding Amaala, whilst I held the hand of a pregnant surrogate, the journey to our complete family. I've never manifested so hard in my life, the vibrations of the sounds 'Sa Ta Na Ma' created such a strong energy around all of us.

By the end of the week, I was re-energised, refuelled. Filled with the belief that soon, we would become parents again. Then, everything changed. As I turned on my phone for the first time since arriving at the retreat, the first message I read was from Ina: 'Kreena, I am so sorry to have to do this in this way. I don't know how to say this, but I can't go ahead with the next journey.'

I couldn't comprehend what was happening. Everything I believed in seemed to come crashing down. My faith that all our adversities had come with their own purpose. My belief that my manifestations would come true. My hopes, my dreams of motherhood seemed to have been taken away from me once again. It was late and I didn't want to call Satty and break the news to him over the phone. I sat on my bed and cried and cried. My best friend, Neelam, walked into the room and found me. I showed her the message and she held me, so tight, as if she were afraid that I would fall if she let go.

I'll never forget that final night on the mountain. I was heartbroken, I was frustrated, I was angry at how dependent I was on other people to make me a mum.

We packed up our bags and headed to the lounge to say goodbye to the friends we had spent the past week with. With each hug came more tears, I didn't share the news with everyone on the mountain, but they could see that something wasn't right – there was no way of hiding it. We digested the news on the flight home and I told Neelam that I would still find a way to bring our embryos to life. If that meant another year on the groups, then that was what I would do. I wasn't ready to give up just yet.

The following morning, I broke the news to Satty. I could see the pain and frustration in his eyes too, we were so close but yet so far. It's in these moments that the pain of infertility and the inability to carry a pregnancy really hit home. When the person you love, the person you envisioned this dream life with, is left hurting because of your inabilities. He had stood by me through cancer, through heart failure, through every single struggle, and I was unable to give him the one thing we both thought we would be able to have without a second thought to any complications.

I spoke to Ina once we were home. I could tell from her message that she was afraid that this would strain our relationship. I wanted to set her straight, to tell her that the negative feelings I was feeling were towards myself, and not towards her. I knew that she didn't owe us a second journey, a part of me knew that nothing was ever guaranteed. I had to remind her that she was the person who made me a mother, to my beautiful, baby girl Amaala, and for that I would always love her and be eternally grateful to her.

The one thing that I had always done since our journey with Amaala was remain within the surrogacy community. I'm so passionate about that – about these relationships being more than baby making. This community is an extension of my friends and family – they've picked me up and given me hope, time and time again.

I spoke to some of my closest friends, many of whom were surrogates. They each came back with the same message: 'Kreena, you are a great intended mother, any surrogate would be lucky to match with you. You will find someone to do this for you, just get back out there'.

So that was what I did. I re-introduced myself on the forums and told everyone of our story, filled with nerves and anxiety. To my surprise, it only took a couple of months to find myself speaking to three different surrogates in more depth. One was a friend made on our first journey, the second a lady from the forums and the third was Laura. Laura was introduced to me by a mutual friend within the surrogacy community.

By October, Laura and I had spoken a fair amount. I could feel some sort of connection, but we needed more time. I was due to travel to India on a charity trek and was afraid that being away would dilute our relationship. When I returned from India, the three surrogates I was speaking to each pulled away for various reasons. Laura messaged to say a new set of intended parents had been in touch and she was due to meet with them.

My heart sank a little, but I shared with her my belief that everything happens for a reason. She shared the same view, and we remained in contact despite that planned meet up. Just a week or so later, she wrote to me saying that things were not going to progress with that couple and that she would love to meet up ahead of Christmas, if we could make our diaries work.

We managed to do just that, and the first time I met

Laura was a dream. We sat and chatted in a tiny little pub for hours on end. Our relationship grew stronger from that date and we arranged to meet again in January, with our families. We shared our views of pregnancy and deal breakers, we began talking about agreements and sharing our thoughts on various points. This moved forward faster than I could have ever imagined, and by mid-January, we were matched and planning dates for a trip to Cyprus. I had anticipated travelling in April, but Laura was keen to travel sooner so that a potential pregnancy wouldn't interrupt her Christmas plans with her children.

Laura is one of the most inspiring women I have ever met. She has created four families through surrogacy and given birth to eight surrogate babies, including ours. She took control of all correspondence with the clinic in Cyprus. She told them her cycle dates and had appointments lined up and ready for scans and blood tests. She took so much pressure away from me, it was incredible to experience and watch her.

By mid-February, we were on a plane and heading out to Cyprus. Two months sooner than I had planned, but my goodness am I glad of that fact. Waiting even one month longer would have meant that COVID-19 would've hit, International borders would have closed and our miracle babies would still be waiting for us in a freezer overseas.

Laura and I checked into our apartment, unpacked our belongings and sat down to a dinner of dippy eggs and toast, perfect! The following morning, we picked up our car rental and drove to the clinic. I'd only been to the clinic and North Cyprus once, to make our embryos, but the place somehow felt like home. We introduced ourselves to reception and were greeted by a member of the team. They took us upstairs and sat us

201

down in the room where Laura would be scanned.

All of a sudden, everything felt so real. These next couple of days could change our lives forever. The scan showed that her lining was looking great, all the medication that Laura had been taking for us had worked a dream. The last of her blood tests were done and then we headed off to explore Kyrenia.

We decided to head to the harbour and find a spot for lunch by the sea. As we arrived, we took a walk and looked out at the fierce waves crashing in front of us. We had lunch at a restaurant built in the middle of the ocean – a window seat gave us the perfect spot to sit, talk and gaze into the distance. That day with Laura was perfect, it gave us time away from our hectic lives in the UK, time to appreciate each other, time to digest all that each of us had been through to get to this point. We headed home by mid-afternoon, armed with a heap of snacks, and settled down for the night with pizza and a film fest of Jurassic Park – Laura's favourite movies!

The following day was transfer day. I woke up early, took a shower then meditated and prayed. We had our breakfast and then drove back to the clinic. After making our final payment and ordering the medication Laura would need when we returned home, we were taken in to see our consultant. He gave us images of the embryos that were going to be transferred into Laura. We had all previously discussed transferring two embryos into Laura and spoke of the likelihood of twins. As a team, we were all always happy for that scenario to play out – for both embryos to take, for a set of non-identical twins to grow inside Laura and join us in our family.

I walked with Laura to the changing room, where she dressed into scrubs. I looked at my phone on the table. The screen was a line of 1s. The time, 1:11pm in

Cyprus and 11:11am in England. I took it as a sign, this was going to work!

I waited patiently outside for Laura. Attempting to read a book but not getting very far due to the constant distraction in my mind. Laura sent a message to let me know the transfer was complete and then sent a picture of the embryos inside her. Tears filled my eyes and my stomach flipped upside down, 'please stick, please stick'.

As we left the clinic that day, we stopped at reception to finalise some paperwork. All being well, we wouldn't have to return again. We turned to leave, and as we did, our doctor was stood behind us. He smiled and said the words: 'One love, two hearts'. I wondered if he was referring to Laura and I as the two hearts, or Laura plus a baby, or maybe two babies? Whatever he was referring to, we could tell that he had a feeling that things were going to turn out well. We collected our belongings and headed off. Laura had always said that she needed salty chips to eat after the transfer, and Google had helped me to locate a Burger King® on our journey home, so we stopped for a late lunch and then returned to our apartment for more Jurassic Park!

Our flight home the next day was fairly uneventful, we sat and chatted, we exchanged photos, and as we got to our cars at Gatwick, we held each other tight for a few minutes before parting company. We hadn't spoken about when we would test but I knew from experience that Laura would probably start peeing on sticks within a week!

We kept in touch daily once we were back. Laura kept me up to date on the medication I needed to order for her and asked what I would like to see on a pregnancy test and when I would want to see it. I was happy to wait for our official test date, but if there was a clear positive before that, then she could let me know.

A couple of days later, I was at my mum's house. She was blissfully unaware that we had even found a match in Laura, or a donor, let alone had any idea of our trip to North Cyprus. It was then that Laura said she was sending through some holiday snaps. I was in the kitchen and decided to look at them once I had sat down with a cup of tea. Twenty minutes later, my jaw hit the floor. The very last image she sent through was of FIVE positive pregnancy tests. Laura had started testing from 4dp5dt (4 days post 5-day transfer) and a faint line could be seen. By 5dpt, that line was much darker, and the digital pregnancy test read '1-2 weeks' pregnant. I couldn't quite believe it – how had we been so fortunate? How had this worked the first time round?

Before I was married, I'd always romanticised about falling pregnant naturally and sitting on the bathroom floor with my husband, waiting excitedly to see two lines pop up. Holding each other the moment we discovered we were pregnant, the way you see it in the movies. I never expected to find out I was pregnant via photos sent on WhatsApp, but that became our reality. Both times, I knew before Satty and it was then my job to make this as memorable for him as I possibly could, to make good of the situation we found ourselves in.

As with Ina and Amaala, I spent that afternoon rushing out to the shops and putting together a memory box and surprise gift for Satty. A baby grow, photos of the tests and a letter board were in the box. As he returned home from work, I sat Amaala down on the sofa with the box and the board. It read: 'BIG SISTER DUTY BEGINS, NOVEMBER 2020'. He wasn't expecting to find out so early and was filled with joy at the news. We celebrated that evening and sent lots of happy pictures to Laura.

As the next few days passed, we compared each of Laura's tests with Ina's from two years prior. Laura's lines were so much darker, and the digital tests were reading one week further ahead than Ina's. By day nine, the test line was darker than the control line. We were certain Laura was pregnant and we both wondered if we were expecting twins.

The 25th February 2020 was our official test date. Laura sent images of every pregnancy test she had taken and we were on cloud nine with the results. The following morning, I was in the kitchen when Satty answered my phone. I could hear an urgency in his voice as he spoke. 'It's Laura,' he said as he handed the phone to me. On the other end of the phone, Laura was in tears. She explained how she had been in severe pain, how her shoulder was hurting, how she had called 111 and now found herself on route to hospital, filled with fear of an ectopic pregnancy.

By this time, the UK had heard of its first case of Covid, then the news that a Brighton resident had contracted the virus. Daily updates were being given in my workplace just a few miles away. We were told that people with existing health conditions, particularly cardiac related, seemed to be at higher risk. I had taken the decision to move to permanent home working and to voluntarily self-isolate to prevent any risk of contracting the virus.

However, the fear in Laura's voice on the other end of the phone played over and over in my mind. I told her I was ready to drive up to be with her, she just needed to say the word. She told me she was fine alone for now and would keep me updated. Laura was discharged in the early hours of the morning – the doctors felt an ectopic was unlikely but couldn't be ruled out, and that Laura would be scanned again in a few weeks. A home pregnancy test showed the lines darkening still, which gave us some reassurance. Her HCG levels came in the next day at 1375. Neither of us had ever known such high levels, we both knew this had to be multiples – twins! Laura said she thought they were boys, due to the levels of sickness and mischief they were giving her, I told her I hoped for a girl and a boy to halve the levels of cheekiness for us both!

The following days were a frantic race to get prescriptions sorted and medication over to Laura for the coming months. We had brought a large amount with us from Cyprus, but a few missing items meant that calls back to Cyprus, conversations with London-based pharmacies and conversions of overseas scripts to UK scripts kept me busy. Eventually, we tracked down everything we needed and had the medication couriered over to Laura.

On 6th March 2020, Laura called me after having her follow-up scan. This was the day we were waiting for – the day we could confirm the pregnancy wasn't ectopic and was, in fact, viable. She asked me if I was sitting down, to which I replied 'yes'. A fear rose inside me, was this bad news? Is that why I needed a seat? 'And remember, don't swear ok', she said on the other end of the phone.

The next thing I knew, Laura was telling me that there were THREE babies inside her tummy. That we were expecting triplets! It took a while for that news to digest. I genuinely hadn't even considered the thought that we could possibly be pregnant with triplets. My first emotion was excitement, then an element of fear. Laura went on to ask me to have a think about what we would want to do. She reminded me of a conversation we'd had when we first signed our agreement: 'Three would be too much,' Satty and I had said, 'I'm not sure we would cope'.

What Laura wanted and needed to know was if we would continue with the pregnancy. If we were happy to have three new additions to our family, or if we would be looking to reduce by one or two babies. I told her that I couldn't consider reducing, that these babies were a gift and one that we couldn't wait to welcome home one day, but that I needed to have the same conversation with Satty. She made it clear that she would be happy to carry three, that whilst she knew the pregnancy would be high risk, she had no desire to reduce it whatsoever.

That evening, when Satty returned home, I had laid a surprise out for him on the table. The letter board read: 'Dhiman Party of SIX' and next to it, three tiny bunnies and one larger one, to represent Amaala and her little siblings.

He walked through the door and read the board. His first words were: 'TRIPLETS! NO WAY, SHUT UP'. We then sat down and spoke about the scan and the three tiny hearts in Laura's tummy.

I asked him how he felt about three new babies, if he was ready, if he would want to reduce. 'No way, no way at all. We will cope, we always do.' His words brought tears to my eyes, even now, writing and reliving those moments, my eyes are full. Amaala came running into the room and we held each other, the tightest hug in history.

Just six months earlier, my world fell apart on top of Juicy Mountain. I thought I may never be a mum again. But here we were, being told we were due to be parents again – three times over. My prayers really were answered, the universe certainly did have my back, she just wanted to test how much I wanted this first.

I told Laura that we were all on the same page, that we all wanted to bring these babies to life, and we couldn't wait for our family to double in size. She told me how relieved she was to hear that, how she was so afraid of having to reduce a pregnancy that she didn't want to.

We could see Covid spreading throughout the UK and were afraid of what the future may bring for this pregnancy. We made a decision early on to have another viability scan, to allow Satty and I to meet our babies for the very first time. That day would be the first and only time we saw our babies together, as a team, until the babies were born. We each watched the screen as three tiny blobs appeared. Three heartbeats, all perfectly placed so that we could watch them in awe. My mind was blown, how had this happened, what would the odds have been? Triplets!! After everything we had been through.

The remainder of our pregnancy became a lockdown pregnancy. Our babies were over 100 miles away from us, and we were restricted from seeing them. Laura was being seen by her consultant every two weeks and we kept in touch with calls and messages. Laura was repeatedly told to reduce the pregnancy, that it was too high risk. We spoke about this between ourselves over and over again; we knew it wasn't something we wanted to do. Being so disconnected when it came to our children and the physicians looking after them was difficult. Eventually, Laura switched consultants. It was important that we found someone who was supportive of our journey and the pregnancy, and fortunately, we found that in our new doctor.

I still find it strange that I'm a mum to four children, but have never met the doctors who helped my surrogates through their pregnancies. A part of me wishes I could have been there to hear the conversations, to hear the risks first hand, to be seen as the babies' mother from the point of conception. However, I also know how important it is to trust your surrogate, to allow her to have her own autonomy when it comes to growing babies from their intended parents. It's another of those scenarios where you simply have to make peace with the fact that for this part of the journey, control doesn't reside with you.

By the time our 12-week scan came around, the UK was in lockdown, pregnant mothers were attending baby scans alone, and intended mothers and fathers appeared to be forgotten. I remember the lead up to the appointment. I had been following the news and social media stories on how partners felt about missing out on seeing their babies and supporting their loved ones at scans. I just kept thinking, what about the mother who doesn't even get to attend the scan? The mother who is not only unable to feel her baby in her womb, but who can now not even see that child for a few precious minutes? What of the dads whose wives weren't carrying their babies? In a conventional set up, the partner may not have attended a scan, but they would have been able to see their baby grow, to feel them kick, to make their own connections. For us, none of that was possible and it hurt… it still does.

Being pregnant through surrogacy during a pandemic was so different, so challenging, so far opposite to our pregnancy with Ina. We weren't able to meet up with Laura, we couldn't have the lazy lunches we wanted, time to check in with her in person, to make sure she was ok. To make sure we were all still ok. We never got to feel our babies kick and the only way we could see them move and grow was via video recordings that Laura would send. For a woman who was soon to be a parent to donor-conceived children, the separation was tough, the fear of not connecting ever present.

Fortunately for us, Laura is super human. She grew our babies perfectly, she sent us audios of their heartbeats routinely, she took pictures continuously and played our voices to the babies frequently. She made sure that she did everything she could to keep us involved, to somehow close the gap that the pandemic had forced upon us. She fought for an exception to be made when it came to scans, and for our 20-week scan, I joined Laura in Northampton. It was the first time I had left my house since Covid took over our lives. It was made clear that I was the babies' mother, and that if every other mother in the country could be there for their children, then I should be allowed to be too. The hospital accepted.

I was quite afraid that day. I knew my health made me vulnerable to coronavirus, but I also knew I couldn't pass up the opportunity to see our three, beautiful babies growing inside Laura. The night before the scan, I prepared everything I would need. A packed lunch and drink so I wouldn't have to stop anywhere on route. A change of clothes for when I was done at the hospital. A face shield, a mask and anti-bac in every form.

Laura was waiting for me in the car park. I didn't know what to do when we first met, instinct said hug her, but Covid said, maybe not. We hugged; a long hard hug. I looked at her bump – my three children, quietly nestled away inside. It was the first time I had seen our baby bump, my eyes filled with tears. Laura took my hand and placed it on her stomach. Everything felt so real. Up until now, our only contact had been remote – no physical touch, no narrowing of the gap between me and my children – but on this day, I was as close as I could be and my heart was as full as it could be.

As we entered the room, I sat to Laura's side, full of excitement to see my babies. The sonographer started the scan and Laura helped her to identify each of the babies. They pointed out organs, limbs, their brains. Everything was so tiny, yet so perfect. I couldn't help but feel like an outsider in the room again. I wished it was me that the cold jelly was hitting, wished it was me pointing out babies one, two and three, me growing them all to life. But that's a dream that I've had to let pass, one that will always remain unfulfilled, but one that I have learnt to make peace with.

Laura and I were each given images of the scan to take home. As we returned to our cars, I opened my envelope and stared down at our triplet babies. I wondered what sex they may have been (we'd chosen not to find out). I wondered when I would see them again, when we would see Laura again. That evening, after sharing everything about my day with Satty, we decided to book a private scan. A scan that would allow Satty to meet his children the following month.

In the weeks before this scan, we had decided to share news of our growing family with our loved ones. As with Amaala, I had chosen to keep some parts of the pregnancy a surprise. So we met outdoors, socially distanced with various family members, and took my trusty letter board with us.

For each reveal, Amaala would show the board. It read: 'BIG SISTER TO BE' and the bottom half of the board was covered with a piece of paper. As we watched the smile grow on the faces we shared this with, the paper was removed and the word 'TWINS' appeared with two scan photos side by side. Those moments were heart-warming and special, memories that we would cherish forever. Life was heavy at the time, everyone was struggling with lockdown, and life with Covid. Sharing our news brought so much joy to everyone. I documented each reveal and shared them with Laura, showing her how happy she was making us all.

The following month, Amaala, Satty and I all travelled to Northampton for our private scan. We felt this could be the last chance we would have to see Laura and the babies, so decided to make it a family affair. Amaala and I waited in the car whilst Satty went in with Laura. I couldn't wait for him to see the babies, to see their arms and legs all tangled together, to hear their little hearts beating. I joined Laura afterwards and then, when the scan was complete, we decided to take a walk in the park together.

That day, we took photographs that went on to be the last ones we would have with Laura pregnant. The last time we would see our babies inside her tummy; the last time Amaala would point to our bump and say: 'Babies in Lauala's tummy'.

A month later, I received a call at 3:45am on 23rd August 2020. 'Kreena, the babies are coming. I'm in an ambulance on my way to hospital'.

I woke Satty up immediately. We called his mum who came over to look after Amaala and within 15 minutes we were on the road, ready to be by Laura's side. The drive to Northampton seemed to take forever. I grabbed my birth plan and checked all the details. I reminded Satty that we were only at 30 weeks, we calmed each other down and prayed that everyone would be ok.

We arrived at Northampton General Hospital at 6am and ran to the delivery suite foyer. I explained who we were and pulled out our birth plan. The lady behind the desk lacked any form of compassion.

'Who are you to the babies and to Laura?' she asked over and over. Then she went on: 'Have you been Covid tested?'

'No,' I replied, 'but neither has Laura – no one knew we would be coming here today.'

After an age of arguing, I asked her to allow a phlebotomist in – a private company who were due to stem cell harvest for us.

'The placenta isn't available, it's been sent away.'

It took a while for the penny to drop. I looked at her, then at Satty. 'Are you telling me the babies are here already?' I cried.

'Did you not know?' she replied.

And that was how we found out our babies had been born – in a hospital foyer, in the middle of a row with a member of staff who had no compassion for our circumstance.

I asked her if all three of the babies were ok and how Laura was getting on. We had no idea at this point that Laura had been rushed in for an urgent c-section.

'I can't tell you anything further,' she went on. 'I shouldn't have told you they were here.'

Satty and I cried, we held each other tight. Every bit of planning was thrown out of the window, and a pandemic kept us away from our babies. We had no idea if all three were alive, we didn't know their sex, we didn't know a thing.

'Can you Covid test us now, please?' we asked.

'No,' she replied. 'We're quite busy.'

It was now gone 7am and we had been waiting in reception for over an hour. It had been over three hours since Laura rang me.

'Why don't you come back at 11am, things will be quieter by then,' she continued. 'Go to McDonalds® for a coffee or something.'

Anger rose inside me – would any other mother or father be asked to sit in a fast food restaurant when their babies had just been born? Not just any baby either: THREE babies, 10 weeks premature. I've since heard stories of disparities in care when it came to pregnancy and birth in the pandemic. How people of colour have been found to have received a poorer level of care. I wonder now if our skin colour was the reason we were treated differently to every other person who became a parent on that day. What other reason was there for my husband, the babies' biological father, to be forced to wait 12 whole hours before he met his children?

We were broken. I messaged Laura to let her know we were on the other side of the door, but she was getting some much-needed rest. We turned to walk away when another nurse stopped us and simply said: 'I just want you to know, all three of your babies are alive, they're well and in Neonatal ICU. Laura had a section and is resting.'

Relief flooded over us, frustration still present, but we walked out knowing we were parents to three little babies.

At around 7pm that night, after twelve hours of waiting, we finally got to meet our babies. Our first stop had been to Laura, to see how she was, to hear of the birth and most importantly, to ask her the sex of the babies. We sat with her, chatted, hugged and hugged some more. She held my hand and told me we had three boys. I was floored, the tears were uncontrollable. None of us had ever imagined three little boys would grace our family. Laura had been alone for the birth. Things moved very quickly and once the babies were here, Covid test restrictions meant no one was allowed to be with her.

We invited Laura to join us as we headed up to see the boys, but she reminded us that these were our children, and it was our moment. She said that if she felt up to it, she would join a little later.

As we walked up to NICU, my stomach was in knots. I had no idea what to expect. We were greeted by the most amazing team. They immediately treated us as the boys' parents. They told us everything there was to know about their birth and the machines that they were each using to stay alive. The consultant quickly followed us into the room and opened with the words: 'You must be Mum and Dad, come and meet your miracles.'

I cried so much – even typing those words today moves me. After all the arguments and frustrations of the day, this man – the man who'd delivered our babies – saw, knew and acknowledged us as their parents.

Satty went to one side of the room and I went to the other. We gazed through the Perspex® boxes – it was like a scene from the movies. These tiny, fragile little babies, perfectly formed, peacefully sleeping. The team told us not to be afraid of the wires or machines, that they looked worse than they were. For some reason, they didn't seem to bother me, maybe because we were so familiar with hospitals. I knew from the moment I met my sons that they would each make it out of NICU, that all they needed was time, love and care.

We washed our hands again, put on gloves and aprons, and opened the incubators of each baby, one at a time, laying our hands on their heads and their stomachs. Feeling how tiny they were in the cup of my hand was mind blowing. Satty and I rotated around the room, making sure no one was left out. We didn't have names picked out, so referred to them as babies One, Two and Three.

One and Two were identical twins, first Aanav then Arvaarn, baby Three was our singleton, Anaayan. One of the nurses asked if I wanted to help change Arvaarn's bedding. I agreed, although I was full of nerves to pick him up. She taught me how to hold him without catching any wires, and on her say so, I picked up my tiny 3lb baby and marvelled at his magnificence.

We left NICU later that evening, and headed home. We kept tight lipped about having three babies and called our families to tell them our 'twins' were boys and were doing well.

The next morning, we were up at the crack of dawn and back on the road. We spent more time with the boys and held each of them between us. Anaayan was the first baby I had skin-to-skin contact with. He was the largest of the three boys, which feels ironic as he is now the smallest. Laura had come up with us on day two, she took photos as I sat with Anaayan, clad in my PPE, my hands never truly touching his, my smile never visible.

As the days passed in NICU, we learned more about how to care for the boys. I watched intensely as the nurses would tube feed them, taking in every step so that eventually I could do it myself. Every day we would wake up, leave Amaala at home and do the 4-5 hours round trip of driving. We would sit with the boys for as long as we could, before making sure we were home ahead of Amaala's bath and bed routine. Each day, we would tell Amaala that her brothers were here, that Mummy and Daddy had to go and look after them. We showed her pictures to help her understand that she was now a big sister.

We used the evenings to roll out more surprises, inviting a couple of our loved ones to our back garden for the triplet reveal. A small group of family, all of whom we had told the babies (twins) had arrived, came over one at a time. I faked a gender reveal, hiding three blue helium balloons in a box. As they opened the box, initially they were excited to know we had sons, then as they read the balloons, they saw it: 'Surprise, it's TRIPLETS!' written on the front. Those reactions were just incredible; the shock and disbelief out of this world.

As time passed, we knew that the daily drive was impossible to maintain. The boys could be in NICU for up to eight weeks, we were exhausted after three days and Amaala was missing Mummy and Daddy very much. We made a decision to relocate up to Northampton, to be close to the boys and to allow ourselves the time we needed to have with Amaala. After days of scouring the internet for a reasonably priced rental, we hit the jackpot and found one across the road from the hospital! That weekend we packed our bags, took all our essential spices and foods, and got ourselves ready for the move. Satty's mum was joining us, so that she could stay with Amaala and be an all-round superstar, prepping all meals, keeping the flat tidy and organising all of us! My baby shower was scheduled for the Sunday before our move. We decided to let it go ahead and use it as an opportunity to let everyone know of the boys' arrival.

Once we moved to Northampton, things began to settle for us all. We quickly formed a routine: one parent at the hospital for the morning rounds, the other with Amaala for breakfast, we would cross over mid-afternoon, with one of us then seeing the boys into the evening before heading back to the flat. I continued to work whilst the boys were in NICU, to allow me more time with them once they were home.

The teams that cared for the boys in NICU were

exceptional. They knew how tough it was looking after three premature babies, they supported us emotionally and practically. They did anything and everything they could to make life easier for us.

Satty and I took it in turns to hold each of the boys over the first couple of days of their lives, and once we were done, we invited Laura to join us for cuddles. Laura fed the boys with her breast milk for as long as she could. She would express the milk and I would feed it to them.

Whilst our time in NICU was intense and challenging, it came with its rewards. We had more time with Laura than we ever expected, our relationship grew deeper and our connection stronger. She would visit when she could, but it was very clear that the boys were now our responsibility – a responsibility we were proud to take over. Much of the boys' final trimester was spent in NICU. It isn't where anyone plans or wants their babies to grow, but for me, the NICU time was actually a big positive. I often felt that caring for them in their Perspex® boxes was an extension of our pregnancy – a pregnancy we missed out on due to the pandemic. Caring for our sons in the neonatal unit was the closest I would ever get to pregnancy, and I drank in every moment.

After five weeks in NICU, our boys were transferred to our local hospital. They travelled down over the course of four days and each time one of them boarded the ambulance for their first road trip, Laura and I sent them off together, holding each other to save ourselves from falling apart. Aanav was the last of the three boys to transfer to East Surrey Hospital. On the day of his transfer, Laura and Satty registered the triplets' birth and we packed up our flat. We said goodbye to Laura, promised to keep in touch, and headed home to start the next chapter of our lives with the boys.

Once we were home, we did everything we needed to to get the house ready for the boys. We bought all of our last-minute purchases, set our bedroom up ready for the day they would come home and began to envision our life together as a family of six. The boys spent a further three weeks in our local hospital. They each moved out of their incubators, and one by one, slept alongside each other in a cot made for multiples.

Seeing them nestled together, closer than they had been in weeks, was simply beautiful. On the 14th October 2020, they were all discharged together. Satty and I spent a night on the ward with them; we were confident that we could manage their needs. Aanav was being sent home on oxygen so we learnt how to change his nasal cannulas, learnt all we had to about any warning signs of discomfort and then walked out of the ward with our three beautiful babies in our arms.

I remember the moment the boys first came home. We walked into the living room, placed their car seats on the floor, and I broke down crying, uncontrollable sobbing. Satty came over and held me close. We did it, we made it, not just NICU, not just the story of the triplets, but the story of our lives.

From the day we received THAT breast cancer diagnosis, through heart failure, through infertility, through surrogacy, through egg donation. Together we made it; together we did it. Somehow, we created this family of six. Our happily ever after.

As I write these words, the boys are now six months old. Raising them has been testing and rewarding all at the same time. From 1.5kg babies, they have grown to a whopping eight kilos. From the sleepy, quiet preemies they were, they have grown into loud, cheeky, happy, smiley babies. From a life away from Mummy and Daddy, to a life by our side, every single day.

Amaala is about to turn three. She is a wonderful big sister; a kind, gentle and loving soul. She spreads joy wherever she goes and makes my heart constantly burst with pride.

Amaala is starting to understand that Mummy's tummy was broken and that she was grown in Ina's tummy, that her brothers were grown in Laura's tummy, but now we all live together and we are a family. She understands that Mummy was once very sick, and that she spent a lot of time at the hospital, but that Mummy is better now, and that Mummy never plans to go back there or to leave her.

I tell her stories about it all, and as the boys grow, I will tell them the same stories too. Because this is how they came to be, these are the obstacles that Mummy and Daddy overcame to build our family. I want them to be proud of it all – of the women who carried them in their wombs, of the donor who gave us the gift of her eggs to create new lives. I want them to know how much they were loved by every person involved in their journeys.

And along the way, I want them, and this story, to inspire others. To give hope to those who find themselves reading this book, looking for comfort, looking for a voice to resonate with their pain.

I am the only South Asian woman I know who has conceived using donor conception and become a mother through surrogacy – there must be more of us out there, more of us who are looking for someone to connect to. I hope that in time, I find that community, and that together we reduce and break down the stigmas that are associated with alternate routes to motherhood.

It doesn't matter what road you take, all that matters is that you choose the one that is right for you. I hope that in reading this journey you're inspired to break convention, to do all you need to to fulfil your dreams, whatever they may be.

All my love, Kreena.

Connect with me on Instagram: @kreenadhiman

Chosen charity

Our charities are CoppaFeel!:
coppafeel.org

They're a breast cancer awareness charity, based in London. They focus on promoting early detection of breast cancer by encouraging women under 30 to regularly check their breasts.

And Future Dreams:
futuredreams.org.uk

They raise funds to support women through their breast cancer journey. They work on a number of campaigns to create awareness and fund research projects, with a main focus on secondary breast cancer.

Ellie and Mark

After three years of TTC and months of medication, they conceived via ICSI and had a baby boy in January 2019. Their journey talks about their experience with diminished ovarian reserve, ICSI and pregnancy after IVF.

Ellie

My story starts in May 2013. I was a 31-year-old single, working girl. After a few failed relationships, I saw an advert for the London Women's Clinic and decided to give them a call to look into having my eggs frozen.

Time was flying and who knew when Mr Right would come along. I went into that meeting full of confidence. Although I smoked at the time and was out most weekends with my friends, I really didn't think that when I decided the time was right, I would have any difficulties conceiving. But just to be on the safe side, why not have eggs frozen?

My mum came along to the appointment with me. I remember the doctor explaining the process and deciding that first, bloods needed to be done, but it shouldn't be too much of an issue. Bloods were taken and I went on my merry way. A week later, a letter dropped on my doormat with the results – my AMH levels were 0.6ng/ml, which was classed as very low. I was devastated. It felt like that was that; I would never be a parent.

I'm the first to admit that after that news, I went on a bit of a mad one. However, in December 2013, I met my now-husband, Mark, and life seemed to take a better turn. That was until we began trying to conceive.

Mark is from a large family and at the time we were TTC, there were an average of two pregnancies a year in the family… none were ours. Why? Why not us? I knew my AMH levels were low but not impossibly low. My husband was healthy, neither of us drank at the time, so why weren't we pregnant? Every announcement was gutting, not because I wasn't happy for them, but why wasn't it us? It is a feeling that every couple TTC will tell you, and only those who have gone through it will know – that feeling of being happy and sad all at the same time.

In 2017 I made 'the call', the one to the GP to start the ball rolling. It lasted all of two minutes: 'How can I help you today, Mrs Casizzi?', 'My husband and I have been trying to conceive for just over a year with no success', 'Ok, I'll refer you to gynaecology, goodbye'. That was it; that was all they had. Deciding not to dwell on it, we waited for an appointment.

A couple of months later, we had our appointment. First things first, the nurse asked me if the GP had carried out any blood tests, which they had not, so my first appointment was a let-down because without those results, there was nothing more to discuss. I left feeling totally deflated. I think deep down, I'd pinned so many hopes on that first appointment, but it was merely an opening discussion and a sign of things to come. I had the bloods done then had to wait weeks for my next appointment.

When my second gynaecology appointment came around, it was decided that I should have a HyCoSy (Hysterosalpingo Contrast Sonography) to check for any blockages in my fallopian tubes and the cavity of my uterus. All came back clear. I have to say, in my case, this was not the most pleasant examination, even though I was told it should be painless.

Given that the HyCoSy came back clear, the decision was then made to place me on a drug called Clomid®, which essentially helps you ovulate by tricking your body into increasing your FSH levels. Initially, I was told to take Clomid® for six months, however this got extended to eight months. By this point, I was becoming increasingly frustrated as I felt that things were just not progressing.

Once I had finished the eight months on Clomid® with no success, they decided to refer me to Guy's and St Thomas' ACU (Assisted Conception Unit). I was told there was no actual wait for treatment but the process of requesting funding from my local CCG could take months. Again, this felt like a kick in the gut – you follow the rules, tick all the boxes, feel like the end is in sight and they throw you another curve ball.

I live in Kent, England and at the time, funding given by my local CCG was as follows: 'Eligible couples requiring IVF, with or without ICSI, will have available to them a maximum of four embryo transfers, including no more than two transfers from fresh cycles'.

I do know that in 2019, Mark and I attended Kent and Medway CCG's consultation on Assisted Conception, as at the time they were looking to cut the above funding to save money. I believe that due to COVID-19 this has now been delayed.

Once we'd been referred by our local hospital to Guy's, the whole process was out of our hands and we could only hope that things would go our way. A few weeks later, I received a call from Guy's hospital advising that funding by my local CCG had been refused. I was gutted to say the least and all I could think was, 'What now?'.

It later turned out the reason for rejection was that

my husband was not registered at the same GP as myself. There ensued a mad dash to my GP to have him register – I literally begged the secretary (who initially said six weeks for registration) to push it through ASAP, explaining that our funding was hanging in the balance. Another wait, or so I thought… the very next day, the secretary called and told me she had pushed it through and wished us luck. I honestly could not believe it! I called Guy's, told them the outcome and a few days later, our CCG agreed the funding and we had our first appointment booked. For a process that had been going on for what seemed like a lifetime, after over two years of waiting, we finally had an appointment!

Appointment day could not come fast enough. I was a ball of nerves and did not know quite what to expect. We made our way to the 11th floor of Guy's & St Thomas' hospital. Now, for those who have never been, I must say it probably has one of the best views of London! That aside, we were both nervous, anxiously waiting our turn. We were called in and the doctor explained both long and short cycles, an internal scan was performed, both of us were sent off for bloods and the next thing we knew, we were sat in front of a nurse explaining to us that I would be on the long protocol and my treatment would start in two days, because of where I was in my current cycle! I remember the words, 'no time like the present'. It was a whirlwind and my mind was racing. I vaguely remember being told how to do the injections but thank god, for once, my other half was paying attention – it also helped that he had previously trained as a midwife!

Before I knew it, we were making our way home with a set of instructions and even more nerves than when we went in. After all the waiting, this was it! It was happening and it was happening fast.

Let me just say this… I don't do needles. I have never liked needles – I mean, why would you willingly allow something to pierce your skin and cause you pain? I am terrible enough when it comes to blood tests but injecting meds daily… let's just say Mark ended up doing every single one, with me kicking and screaming. By the time the trigger shot came along, after 23 days of injections (36 injections in total) my lower abdomen was beyond tender. I was bruised, and frozen peas had become my new best friends, BUT we'd made it to egg collection relatively easily and I hadn't really had any side effects to the drugs. It was all on track.

My Ovitrelle® shot (trigger shot) was to be given at 1am, exactly 36 hours prior to egg collection. We must've set six or seven alarms to make sure we didn't miss it. I have never seen my husband run down the stairs so fast when that alarm went off. Once it was done, it was all systems go for collection.

I will never forget that day, walking through the double doors and being prepped for the procedure. Mark was called away to do his part as I was being wheeled into theatre. There was a team of maybe five or six people, and I said to the anaesthetist, 'Just hit me with a sledgehammer, no heroes here', and that they did. I remember waking up and looking out the window at the view across London and being offered tea and biscuits. It was done. It was out of my hands and I had to put all my faith in the medical team to know what they were doing.

Once fully conscious, the embryologist came into my cubicle. They had retrieved 17 eggs but there was a slight issue – Mark's sample was not what they were expecting. Rather than classic IVF, they were going to have to go with the option of ICSI – which is where sperm is injected directly into the egg to hopefully increase fertilisation rates. Luckily, this was covered by our local CCG, but had it not been, we would've had to find £1000 there and then.

I saw Mark's face and I knew he was not feeling good. I knew this had come as a shock and that he was blaming himself, but none of us could have predicted this – we were prepped, the tests had been done, yet nature was throwing us another curve ball.

They told us to go home, rest up and they would call the next day to tell us how things were going. The wait: it is a killer. I am not patient, never have been. I had to learn the hard way.

It. Felt. Like. Forever!

Finally, my phone rang: 17 eggs collected, 10 mature ones that were injected, nine fertilised, now to wait. Yep, it doesn't end there, now we had to wait to see if our embryos would make it to blastocyst.

I eventually got the call: embryo transfer was happening on day 5. This was it, responsibility was back to me. We walked in and I remember the nurse pulling out a Petri dish. This was our one good embryo – unfortunately, the others just weren't advancing as they should. This was our one shot.

The doctor transferred the embryo into my womb and the sonographer pointed out to me this tiny little dot on the screen and said, 'That's your baby'. It was the strangest moment: happiness, excitement, anxiety, you name it, all running through my body. Strangely, Mark was humming 'You are my sunshine', which I believe was a nervous hum as it's never happened since. And just like that, it was done!

But I didn't just leave it there… oh no, I had a stupid moment. I was desperate for the toilet (for the embryo transfer you need a full bladder) and in the craziness of the moment, I said, 'If I go to the toilet, will it fall out?'. The doctor looked at me like I was crazy and replied: 'We placed the embryo in your womb, not your bladder, but just so you know, you're not the first to ask that'.

I was given discharge paperwork with a test date I will never forget: 17/05/2018 – the 15-year anniversary of the passing of my uncle, with whom I had a very close relationship. I only hoped that he would be looking down on us and make it happen.

We went home and so began the two-week wait. I kept myself unbelievably busy! I didn't stop because stopping meant thinking and I did not want to think. Our circle of people in the know was small. In the middle of the wait, we had a family wedding. Rather than get a hotel room, I decided to drive (easier to explain the not drinking). One of the only people who knew, my sister-in-law, asked me how I was feeling. She wanted to know how I was coping and explained that she wouldn't be able to do it, she would have to know. I just remember looking at her and saying, 'Because I don't think about it!'. And that was as far as I would allow the conversation to go.

The night before my test date, Mark was in the bath and I had an early morning, so I said to him, 'I will do one of the hospital tests, probably won't say anything as it's not the first urine of the day but whatever, I'm intrigued'. At this point, I'd had no signs either way and I live by the motto: hope for the best, expect the worst. I took the test and it immediately, without hesitation, showed positive. It was crazy! It was so quick, in fact, that my husband tried telling me I had done the test wrong. There's only one way to pee on a stick!

We called our parents under strict instructions that no one, not a soul, was to be told. The next morning

229

(official test day), I took another test and as expected, it was positive. So, after informing the clinic, we waited patiently for our 8-week scan.

During the wait, I carried on with the pessaries. Yes! What they fail to tell you is that on top of all the injections, the internal scans, the egg collection, and embryo transfer, there are those pesky pessaries. The ones that you either insert vaginally or rectally. Progesterone. Very important but not the nicest thing to do, twice daily or more, until 12 weeks of pregnancy. I mean, let's be honest, by the time this process is over, more people than you can imagine will have seen your bits and all dignity will have gone out the window.

Our 8-week scan came around and I had a 'Rachel' moment (you know, Rachel from Friends). Mark, having trained as a midwife, was all over the scan like a rash. He knew exactly what he was looking for and at – me on the other hand, no idea. Both my husband and the sonographer said, 'Can you see your baby?' and I replied, 'Yes'. They started chatting and I finally had to confess that I did not have a clue what I was looking at.

After the scan, we were fully discharged from the clinic and handed over to our local midwifery team. You'd think after all that things would go smoothly but no, my pregnancy was a non-stop emotional rollercoaster from start to finish.

At 10 weeks, I had a bleed and was taken to the EPU at my local hospital. It was terrifying, but thankfully we were given the all clear. We then had our 12-week scan and the baby was growing well. I was asked if I wanted the usual screening tests done for Down's syndrome, Edwards' syndrome and Patau's syndrome. I thought nothing of it and agreed.

We went home and planned to have our family

round that weekend to announce our news. The day before we planned to tell our families, I was at work and I felt wet, really wet. I had just been to the toilet so it could not be that. I rushed to the toilet and all I could see was blood. It was everywhere. I was supposed to be going for lunch with my colleagues, but instead, I jumped in a cab and went to the EPU at St Thomas' hospital.

I just remember the nurse asking me if I had a pad and me saying I did not, as I didn't think I needed one. I sat there for what felt like a lifetime; Mark came from work and we waited.

Finally, we were called in for a scan and there was our little fighter, jumping around, not a care in the world. They had no idea why I was bleeding but said, 'it happens'. Relieved, we told our families that weekend. It was finally hitting home that it was happening – we were finally making our announcement and we could not be happier.

A few days later however, I got the results from my screening tests and it came back with a very high probability of Down's syndrome. The options I was given were as follows:

- Continue with the pregnancy without taking things any further, but that would mean I would have a specialist team at the birth just in case.

- Have an amniocentesis performed but that was not without risk, and given the two large bleeds I'd had, not advised.

- Private DNA testing at a cost of £300 (although I believe this is now available on the NHS)

- A termination

I spoke to my husband and we decided that either way, we wanted to know, so we opted for the private DNA test. I understand this was not something that everyone could have afforded there and then so we were lucky in that respect. I also understand that every person's reaction to the test results is different – we chose to do what we felt was right for us at that time.

I booked the appointment and a couple of days later, headed to the Wolfson Institute in London for my blood test. Basically, they count the number of chromosomes in my blood sample. They know that I don't have 21, so when counting, if they find an extra 1, then they know this is coming from the baby.

Our test results came back negative for Down's syndrome, and the results were transferred to my local hospital to be kept on record if I ever fell pregnant again. They could compare their results of a fresh pregnancy to my DNA results and not national averages.

After all the ups and downs of emotions, we had hoped the rest of the pregnancy would be as smooth as possible. However, at around the 6-month mark, whilst babysitting our niece and nephew, I didn't feel quite right. I had bad cramps. I left Mark to watch the kids and took myself home (I did not want to ruin my sister-in-law's birthday for something that was probably nothing). I drove right by the hospital thinking, should I go in?

I did not and I went home. Later, I called the midwife, who advised paracetamol and sleep and if it was still bad in the morning to go in. The next morning, I felt ok but by the afternoon, I was in agony. Mark called the midwife, and I was told to go in for a check-up. They carried out bloods, which came back normal. The midwife had a feel of my tummy and when she did, I cried out in pain. She then performed an ultrasound and thought that the baby had pierced the lining of the womb.

The obstetrician was called (a rather good looking one, when I was not looking my best) and concluded that I had a fibroid on the outer lining of the womb, which was becoming bigger and more aggravated as the baby grew, but there was nothing they could do.

After that, my pregnancy progressed at a somewhat normal pace. We hit our due date of 18th January 2019 and there was absolutely no sign of movement. I had a midwife appointment and she asked if I would like a sweep. I agreed, at this point I'd take anything to bring on labour. In my experience, it was painful and achieved nothing. Another appointment was scheduled a few days later.

At my next appointment, given that there was absolutely no movement from baby, it was decided to schedule an induction for 12 days over. In my case, 30th January. I was told it could take anywhere between 24-72 hours (in some cases longer), and that this would not be a quick process.

In the days that followed, I tried just about every old wives' tale to kick start labour but this baby was not budging. On the 30th, Mark and I drove to the hospital, ready for the long process of induction. On the way there, his brother texted to wish us luck and signed off by saying, 'remember, the delivery room is like a war zone' – in my case, he couldn't have been closer to the truth.

We arrived at midday and the pessary to induce labour was given around 2:30pm. By 4pm I was climbing the walls. After this point, I only remember snippets of what was happening around me and have had to rely on my husband and my mum, who were present at the birth, to fill in the gaps.

I did not have the best experience for my birth. My midwife was a large part of the outcome. Now, not everyone has the same experiences (and no births are the same), and I honestly can say that in 99% of cases midwives do an amazing job, unfortunately for me that wasn't the case. I felt that I wasn't listened to. I knew what my body was telling me to do and no matter how many times I said, 'I need to push', she wouldn't believe me – even at one point saying I didn't know what I was talking about.

My labour went very fast for a first labour (and an induction at that), from start to finish it was 3 hours 58 minutes. Had it not been for the swift actions of a more senior midwife, who took over and without even checking me said I needed to be transferred to delivery immediately, there was a strong possibility the outcome could've been very different. As it was, our beautiful baby boy was born at 19:58 on 30th January 2019, weighing in at a hefty 8lb 4oz.

He will forever be our one in a million. IVF is not an easy solution as some may wish to portray – it is a necessity, not a choice, and it's not something I would wish upon anyone.

I often felt throughout our journey that it was something that should be kept private, not to be talked about, however since having my son, I have become so passionate about raising awareness. Since sharing our experience, I have had friends come to me asking for advice. Ones who have been struggling behind closed doors with infertility, trying to navigate their way through not just the emotional toll, but the medical side of things too – where to go, who to speak to, it's a minefield.

It takes a strong woman to give birth to a child, but I believe it takes an even stronger one to give birth to an IVF baby.

We've decided that our story doesn't end here

though. Whilst writing about our journey for this book, Mark and I were quietly undergoing another ICSI cycle, in the hope of giving our son a sibling. Unfortunately, after a relatively straightforward treatment process, we lost both of the embryos that had been transferred. We still remain hopeful that we can try another cycle in the future.

Chosen charity

Our charity is Fertility Network UK:
fertilitynetworkuk.org

They provide information, advice, support and understanding for those dealing with infertility.

Alana and Amanda

$100,000 spent
1251 days
14 failed attempts
11 embryos transferred
5 IVF stim cycles
5 chemical pregnancies
4 years TTC
4 surgeries
2 pregnancies
1 reciprocal IVF cycle
1 rainbow baby on the way

Alana

We are Alana and Amanda, a same sex couple from Sydney, Australia.

I met Amanda in 2012, when we were set up by a good friend of ours, and it was one of those love at first sight moments – we knew we were meant to be. Amanda assumed she would never have children because she was gay and she didn't want to carry a child herself. Before I met Amanda, I had started looking into single motherhood by choice options for having a child. Having a child was really important to me and I didn't know when I would meet the right person to start a family with.

We talked about having children early on and the plan was always that I would carry the child. I was ready from day one but it took Amanda a little more time to come around to the idea. We decided to have some time together first, so we travelled, had fun and bought a house. When our first niece was born in 2016, Amanda fell in love and knew it was time for us to start trying for a baby.

We saw a fertility specialist at the end of 2016, as we chose to have treatment through a fertility clinic and use a de-identified clinic donor, as opposed to finding our own donor or doing at-home inseminations. We both had all the standard tests and everything came back normal. In a follow-up appointment with the doctor, I told her that I thought I would have trouble conceiving, as that's what I'd always been told by the doctor who managed my PCOS diagnosis from my teenage years. This doctor laughed at me and told me I would easily fall pregnant because the only reason I was at the clinic was for donor sperm. I felt reassured that everything would be ok. We started off with IUIs, as I was only 'socially infertile' and not medically infertile and wasn't able to access the rebates for IVF.

In June 2017, we picked our top five donors (we found out the night before the IUI which donor we had – we were told it was very rare not to get your first or second pick) and started our first IUI cycle. On a cold winter morning in June, I went in for my very first blood test and scan of the cycle. The doctor didn't have the greatest bedside manner and told me to drop my pants and sit down, while they stayed in the room – it was a very rude shock to the world of fertility treatments. I was told by the doctor that my lining wasn't ready yet and sent for my blood test.

This doctor took on a lot of patients and staff were stretched thin. The nurses called that afternoon in a panic because I needed to do my trigger shot NOW! I didn't understand, as the doctor had told me I wasn't ready but I trusted that the medical professionals knew better than I did, even though my gut told me it wasn't right. It was cycle day 11 and I went in for my first IUI.

I still remember that first two-week wait. We hadn't told anyone what we were doing, apart from a set of friends who went to the same clinic. A few days in, we couldn't handle the wait any longer and called our mums to tell them. We called my mum first and she just said, 'Ok, no worries. Hang on, let me just go upstairs and see if I can find it'… she got to her bedroom and closed the door and squealed, 'OMG! That is so exciting!' – she had people over at the time, so had to go back downstairs and act normal. Unfortunately, it was a negative on test day.

The second IUI was a disaster and had to be cancelled. We picked our top five donors, it was déjà vu with the blood tests and scans, then at cycle day 11, I was again told to do the trigger shot, and then we got the call that none of our top five donor choices were available. I have never been so stressed in my life! We had a look at the list again and picked a few others, who were also not available because the list that was meant to be updated weekly hadn't been updated for a month. We had 2-3 choices of donors to pick from, none of which seemed right for us. We cancelled the cycle and had our money refunded. We were furious and devastated, but it didn't seem right to just pick any donor.

At this point, I was starting to lose trust in our clinic, however we continued with IUI three. Again, it was much the same story: an early trigger that didn't feel right and a negative result. We had a meeting with the doctor. I was so upset that all they could say was, 'You can't expect to roll six on a dice every time'. There was no reassurance; there was no advice. I was signed off as medically infertile and we decided we would start IVF, as it seemed like much more of a guarantee.

We started our first IVF cycle in December 2017 – it was very daunting but exciting. I did all the stims over the Christmas break, then triggered on New Year's Day 2018 and had my egg collection on the 3rd January. I got 12 eggs and I was stoked!

The day after, we were at the shopping centre when I got the call with the fertilisation report. Our clinic at the time did ICSI as standard, as we were told it had a much higher success rate. I was told that six eggs fertilised. I was in complete shock – no one at the clinic had really explained the rule of thumb that you lose about 50% at each stage. I thought I had done a lot of reading on IVF but we had high expectations as there was nothing 'wrong' with me. We were so naïve. It took a lot for poor Amanda and our mums to calm me down. I felt like I had failed already.

This clinic only did day 3 transfers, I knew other clinics did day 5 transfers, but again, I kept telling myself that I needed to trust the doctor. Day 3 came and we went in for our first fresh transfer – we were so excited. Seeing our little embryo on the screen hit me hard, I didn't think I'd get that emotional, and still to this day, every time I see my embryos for the first time my eyes well up – it's an incredible feeling.

It felt like so much more was at stake in this TWW because the IVF cycle cost so much more than an IUI. I started testing at about 10dpt. I had Pregnyl® boosters so I knew the pregnancy tests would be positive but I wanted to test out the Pregnyl®. I watched the tests get darker and darker, but had no idea if I was pregnant – in hindsight, it was quite obvious! On the 20th January 2018, I had my pregnancy blood test – it was the longest day of our lives. We suspected we were pregnant but really had no idea what to expect.

The nurse finally called around 4pm and said, 'Are you sitting down? Because I have good news! Congratulations, you are pregnant'. She continued talking and I really didn't hear a thing – I was shaking, I couldn't believe it, I had no idea what to do, I could barely think straight. I WAS PREGNANT!

I quickly left work, trying to avoid seeing my dad and brother who I worked with at the time. I called Amanda and all I could say was 'yes' and then I started to cry and laugh at the same time. I drove to an acupuncture appointment sobbing, laughing and saying 'OMG' over and over again.

The first person I told was my acupuncturist. She

hugged me and we both cried together. I got home and walked in the door to see Amanda holding a bunch of flowers for me. We just stared at each other, not knowing what to do. The plan was to visit family over the weekend but Amanda couldn't wait. We drove straight over to my parents' place to tell them. They were, of course, confused as to why we had shown up but no one twigged what we were about to say.

Amanda asked them what they were doing on the 28th September… they stared at us blankly. My mum was standing over the other side of the room, in the kitchen, and my dad, my brother and sister-in-law were sitting in the lounge. Amanda continued with, 'Because that's the day our baby is due!'. I will never forget the squeal Mum made as she ran across the room to hug me. She never shows much emotion and she was so excited. My brother and sister-in-law said, 'Congratulations' and my dad said, 'I think it's too early to be excited, anything could happen'. We were on cloud 9! We were so happy and felt so lucky that IVF had worked first time for us.

We had a scan at 6 weeks and saw the tiny little heartbeat of our baby. It's the most magical experience to see your baby's heartbeat for the first time. My stomach was growing and my body changing, but I was worried that I didn't have any morning sickness at all. Everyone told me I was one of the lucky ones and not to worry. My mum didn't really get morning sickness herself but none of that reassured me.

At 9 weeks, I had another scan booked. The GP told me it wasn't necessary to have a dating scan for an IVF baby but I insisted. The night before, I knew it wasn't going to be good news but I didn't tell Amanda and I didn't sleep that night. The next morning, I was so anxious. We went in for the scan and the technician decided to do a stomach ultrasound first but warned it may be too early to see anything and I may need an internal scan.

As soon as I saw the foetus on the screen, I knew it should have been bigger by now. I watched her quickly put the heartbeat sound on and off but there was no sound, no typical heartbeat line you see. I started panicking. The technician asked me to empty my bladder and come back for an internal scan. I shut the door in the bathroom and tried my hardest to pull it together for Amanda and brace for the bad news. I walked down the hallway, back to the room, and I could see Amanda smiling at me. My heart broke because I thought that she thought everything was going well… but I later found out she was trying to be strong for me.

After a quick internal scan, the technician quickly switched the screens off, turned to us and said those dreaded words: 'I'm so sorry, there's no heartbeat'. I'd had a missed miscarriage – I didn't even know what that meant. I looked at Amanda, who had tears streaming down her face, but I was numb. I had no idea what to do next but the technician was great and instructed us to call my GP and get in ASAP, and if I couldn't, then to go to the local hospital emergency department.

We walked out in complete shock and I fell over and cut my knee. I could feel blood running down my leg but I couldn't care less. I called the GP and they could see me in an hours' time, so we drove to my mum's place to wait. The whole drive there I just kept saying to Amanda, 'I'm not crying, why am I not crying?' – I didn't understand.

As soon as I saw my mum, I broke down. It was at that point it was real. Amanda kept herself busy, telling family and close friends what had happened. She started cancelling appointments that had been booked and cancelling various app and email subscriptions so I wouldn't get any weekly update reminders.

We got to the GP and she was there waiting for us. She was very compassionate and took us through all the options and steps. She had called my fertility clinic and the OBs at the local hospital to let them know what had happened. I opted for a D&C because I just wanted it over. I couldn't bear the thought of waiting for the miscarriage to start naturally.

Our next step was to head to the emergency department at the local hospital. We waited for six hours to see an OB. It was too late for surgery that day so I was booked in for day surgery the next day. We went home, exhausted and devastated, wondering what the hell had just happened. We weren't due to be at the hospital until midday the next day but I had to fast from the night before. It was torture waiting around. I remember every single moment of that drive to the hospital. And all I could think was, 'Why isn't this drive in 7 months' time when I'm in labour?'.

The staff at the hospital were really great with me and put me in a room by myself so we could have our privacy. I had to have a pessary to dilate my cervix and then we waited and waited and waited. We got to the hospital at 12pm and I didn't go into surgery until after 5pm. At this point, I was so hungry and felt so dehydrated. Then things started getting a bit disastrous.

The ward clerk took me down to surgery while I sobbed. I made sure that I told everyone that I wanted the pregnancy contents genetically tested, to try to find out what was going on. The nurses kept ensuring me that the doctor would talk to me before surgery, so to tell him then. The anaesthetist started to get me ready. I told her that there's always trouble getting the canula into my hand but she kept trying anyway. She tried both hands and three different needles and couldn't get it in – there was blood everywhere and I was starting to panic. Finally, the nurse suggested that maybe she try my forearm. It finally worked and I started feeling drowsy. Another anaesthetist walked over and exclaimed, 'WHAT ARE YOU DOING?', to which she responded, 'She's really upset and panicked, so I'm just sedating her now'. Both the nurse and the other anaesthetist said, 'NO, NO, NO! She wanted to talk to the doctor', and she responded, 'It's too late'. I looked at the nurse, panicking, asking her to tell the doctor about the genetic testing… I don't even know if I got a full sentence out before going completely under.

No genetic testing was done. I woke up in a dark room, by myself, and insisted that the nurse call Amanda. It took a while but they reluctantly called her. Amanda helped me up to go to the bathroom. In my state, I wasn't expecting that there would be blood everywhere and none of the hospital staff thought to provide me with any information on what happens after a D&C. We left the hospital with no information and no idea what to expect in the coming weeks of grief. We finally got home at about 9pm.

The next few days were a blur of pain, tears and bleeding. I bled for 10 days and that was such a brutal reminder of what happened. I went back to work four days after surgery, still bleeding heavily, with no one knowing what had happened. The first day back, a lady I worked with brought her new baby into the office to meet everyone. I just had to put on a brave face.

The next few weeks were horrible. There was a lot of pressure from family members to 'move on' and 'just get over it', when we just wanted to be alone and have time to ourselves. People took our reclusiveness as us having an issue with them but we just needed time to grieve. I didn't understand why people couldn't be more understanding and sympathetic. It was a very steep learning curve that people are uncomfortable with grief. I just wanted someone to listen to me, not try and fix the situation.

I got my period back exactly eight weeks after the D&C. In hindsight, I wasn't ready to try again, but I was determined to start again and no one was going to stop me! We had no idea the heartbreak and tough times that lay ahead of us. As soon as my period came back, we jumped into our first frozen transfer. I honestly don't remember anything from that time – I think I was still numb and looking back, we probably should have waited. Needless to say, it was another negative cycle.

In between the next cycles, I went to my sister-in-law's baby shower. My pregnancy was just six weeks behind hers. Why I went, I still don't know because I spent most of the time trying not to cry.

We had one frozen embryo left and at the time, it was really important to us to keep our same donor. When we'd found out we were pregnant, we'd had the option of buying additional vials of our donor sperm for exclusive use. This would mean they were ours to use for future cycles. We'd thought we had time to purchase more and didn't get a chance before the miscarriage. The way our clinic worked, was that once your frozen embryos were gone, you weren't guaranteed the same donor – you had to pick from the list again. I tried my luck and used the loophole that we did have an embryo frozen still. Somehow, I was able to start a new IVF cycle with the same donor.

Our clinic did day 3 transfers as standard but I'd done a lot more research and reading, and insisted on taking the embryos to day 5. The doctor wasn't impressed but agreed. IVF cycle two was the first time I was sold 'add-ons'. I was told these new and exciting cultures that could be added when embryos are developing, gave your embryo a better chance of growing stronger and implanting. I was desperate, and I went for it. The cycle went along normally, from what I believed and knew at the time. It was tough and stressful but I got through it. I had 12 eggs collected, eight were fertilised.

Even though we were insistent on day 5 embryos and a day 5 transfer, we transferred one of our day 3 embryos. It was a Saturday and it made sense at the time to transfer on a Saturday morning and have the weekend to rest. The remaining seven embryos were left until day 5 to develop. Three embryos ended up making it to day 5 and were able to be frozen. The embryo grading system at this clinic always showed my embryos to be fairly standard and definitely not top quality, but I was told this was normal and that grading didn't really mean a lot anyway.

Another two-week wait went by. I suspected it was a negative result again, even though the pregnancy test was positive. I thought it was the medications still in my system. I had my blood test and waited all day for the nurse to call me. When she finally called, she told me that I was 'a little bit pregnant' but the HCG level was very low and the pregnancy wouldn't last. It was called a chemical pregnancy. She rushed through her spiel and finished the conversation as soon as she could. I was so confused, I hadn't thought there was an answer worse than no. What the hell was 'a little bit pregnant'?!

I called Amanda but really wasn't sure what to say. I hadn't asked the nurse questions because it wasn't the

news I was expecting. That night, we called the nurses'
after-hours number and spoke to a different nurse. This
nurse took the time to listen to us and explain what was
going on. We were devastated but at least we had a
better understanding of what was happening.

At this point, we were 12 months in with six failed
cycles. After each failed cycle, we had a WTF phone
call with the doctor, and every time I got the same
analogy, 'You can't expect to roll 6 on a dice every
time'. There was no other advice, no other suggestions
or changes in plans, and I got pretty sick of hearing the
same analogy over and over again, so I decided it was
time for a second opinion.

I researched clinics and doctors, and came up with
one who I thought looked really great and a second who
was high up in the same clinic. I really wanted to
transfer my embryos to their clinic but they wouldn't
accept any embryos from the clinic I was at. Red flag!
The first doctor, who was higher up at the clinic,
basically pushed me away and told me I'd just had bad
luck. They cost a fortune so I wasn't happy that they
were so dismissive of me. The other doctor who I'd
researched actually listened to me and seemed to be the
first professional willing to listen to what I was saying.

I was sent for more tests but assured that it was
probably just bad luck and not to give up yet. I went
back a couple of weeks later for the results and nothing
really showed up as being a problem. The only thing
that stood out was a really low iron level. The doctor
couldn't believe that the other clinic had let me do IVF
with such low iron levels. Their suggestions were to get
an iron infusion and either leave my embryos at the
other clinic and start fresh, or transfer the embryos we
had left, hope for the best and if we weren't successful,
then move to the new clinic.

I was a wreck by this stage. Amanda was heading to Melbourne for a business trip so I decided to take some time off and go with her. I wandered around the city aimlessly for a couple of days, feeling lost. On our last morning, I woke up when the alarm went off and rolled over to look at Amanda. She was already awake and had a strange look on her face. She looked at me, with tears rolling down her face, and told me that our new niece had been born. We were, of course, happy for Amanda's brother and sister-in-law, but we both had an overwhelming sadness that our baby should have been following in six weeks' time. We cried together in bed.

We both dreaded the day we got home and had to visit the hospital. I picked Amanda up from the station and had a panic attack in the car. We walked onto the maternity ward really anxiously and there was a woman on a foetal monitor. The sound of the heartbeat was so triggering that I turned around and walked out. It took me a while to calm down again. We finally worked up the courage to go in and put on a brave face – it was really tough. We stayed for as long as we could and then got out of there. We both got into the car and cried. It was so hard to have these conflicting emotions.

It was now October 2018 and we decided we couldn't just leave our embryos behind. We had four embryos left and our aim was to transfer them all before 2018 was finished and move to a new clinic in 2019 if we had no success – with the best-case scenario being that one of the embryos was successful. Around the same time, I was spending every moment I could researching and reading as much as I could about recurrent implantation failure and started looking into natural killer cells.

For the October cycle, I insisted on trying different medications, a different trigger and progesterone pessaries post transfer. By this point, we were pros at injecting medications but that didn't make a difference and it was another negative.

I was emotionally spiralling out of control. I was angry, I was emotional, I was hard to live with and I wasn't myself. I was determined to get through all the embryos by the end of the year so I started another cycle straightaway, with the hope I'd be pregnant on my birthday.

Our November cycle was hell. And IVF started taking its toll on us physically. Before the cycle started, I was really sick with the flu and then Amanda was scheduled for a day surgery. As we got further into the cycle, it was looking like my embryo transfer could be on the same day as Amanda's surgery. Luckily, it didn't end up that way but Amanda did pick up a nasty virus from the hospital. We were both so run down and so sick. I also had an appointment with a reproductive immunologist just after my transfer. He put me on aspirin, steroids and stronger progesterone pessaries, and straightaway told me, 'You'll be pregnant this cycle so I don't expect to see you back'.

This doctor seemed to be a miracle worker and I was at the point of delusion, so I believed it. I was well aware of my body by now and a couple of days before my pregnancy test, I started getting sore boobs and a pulling feeling in my uterus – the feelings I had only experienced with my pregnancy and chemical pregnancy. I didn't want to get my hopes up though. I did a home pregnancy test and it was faintly positive. I anxiously waited until the next morning to test again and the line had faded. I knew it was another chemical pregnancy. Test day came and I was right: it was another chemical.

We had two embryos left and only one cycle

remaining in 2018. I was determined to start fresh in 2019 so I stood my ground and pushed for two embryos to be transferred, and the doctor agreed. I went back to the reproductive immunologist, who told me my natural killer cells were on the low side of high and I'd need the full immune protocol for my double transfer.

It was December, it was my third back-to-back cycle and I was a crazy, hormonal wreck. I had fights with Amanda, I screamed at my mum for no reason and was very withdrawn. I was a nightmare to be around and everyone walked on eggshells or avoided me. I started on antibiotics, steroids and blood thinners before transfer. I was so worried about putting on weight with steroids but somehow ended up losing weight, even though I was eating everything in sight.

Amanda was really busy at work with Christmas, so this was the first embryo transfer she didn't attend and my mum came with me. After transfer, I was on strong progesterone pessaries and three days before Christmas, I had my first intralipid infusion. It was nine hours of watching white fluid drip into my arm, in an attempt to help implantation. I was meant to be relaxing but I found it impossible; I was so agitated I was jumping out of my skin.

We somehow got through Christmas and then it was my brother's wedding. I started getting the same feelings in my uterus, sore boobs, and faint pregnancy tests. I'd lost hope by now and assumed it was just another chemical pregnancy. We were setting up for my brother's wedding in 40 degree heat and I felt like rubbish. I was cramping and felt like I was getting my period when I got the call to say it was another chemical pregnancy. Once again, we had to put on brave faces during the wedding the next day.

2018 was a rough year but we had hopes for a fresh

start in 2019. We started the year with a new clinic and a new doctor. This new doctor seemed really progressive and thorough. They wouldn't let me start a new IVF cycle until I'd had investigatory surgery. I was booked in for a hysteroscopy and laparoscopy in March, with the plan to start IVF around May/June. Surgery went well and I recovered fine, apart from being a little bit sore from the incisions. I was told by the doctor that there was a second surgeon in the room, who would remove any endometriosis if needed.

I was called with the results the next day. The doctor said there was a little bit of endometriosis on a blood vessel going to the uterus that was too dangerous to remove and 'there might be endometriosis in the uterus, but there might not be, I don't know'. I just remember thinking: 'Hang on, we specifically went in looking for endometriosis and paid a lot to do that, and now I'm getting a maybe answer!'.

The doctor also said my uterus looked inflamed and took a biopsy to send off for testing. They thought I maybe had a uterine infection, that are generally silent in symptoms. I started on strong antibiotics in an attempt to get rid of it. A few days later, the test results were received and there was no infection: 'The inflammation could have just been from where you are in your cycle'. There were no conclusive results and it felt like the surgery had been a waste of time.

Every result was coming back 'normal' and I just wished there was actually something wrong with me that could be worked on. In between surgery, we were picking donors and almost got caught up in a dodgy, South African sperm donor clinic but luckily my gut told me not to go ahead. We had donors message us using my name! We made it to the top of the list for the American donors, where there were only two to choose from. Luckily, one of them was mostly what we were looking for. Previously, we'd put so much emphasis on carefully picking the 'right' donor but by now, we just needed someone healthy who could help me get pregnant. A lot of money later, eight vials of sperm arrived in Sydney.

May came and it was time to start our third IVF cycle. I decided to stick with the reproductive immunologist and do a full immune protocol again. We talked medications and dosages with the new doctor and they decided to keep my dosages high, like the last cycle at the previous clinic. I trusted the new doctor and thought that the higher dosage meant more eggs developing. The doctor also wanted to do ICSI, as that's what I'd done at the last clinic – again, I trusted that it was in my best interest.

This time around, I tried a few different medications. Everything was going along well and it seemed like the doctor was being thorough – I even had to introduce another medication halfway through the cycle. There were about 10-12 follicles, which was similar to previous cycles. After the retrieval, I woke up from surgery by myself and was told only seven eggs had been collected. I was devastated. Amanda couldn't take any more time off work so my mum was on her way to pick me up. I was so upset that Amanda had to leave work and come home with me. I didn't understand how we'd ended up with our worst result yet.

The next day, we got the fertilisation report: only five eggs were able to be used for ICSI and out of the five that were injected, only four fertilised. Our odds were getting smaller and smaller. At this clinic, we were able to log into an app and watch our embryos grow, which was pretty special. At day 3, we had three embryos but one was quite slow and looking like it wouldn't make it. It was the first time I wasn't sure if we'd have any embryos to transfer.

On day 5, we went in for transfer and we were both so anxious. I was convinced that we weren't going to have any embryos. Finally, the embryologist came to see us and told us that we had two hatching blastocysts. We went into the transfer room and they put the embryo up on the screen; the embryologist talked to us about the hatching blastocyst. At the previous clinic, we'd been told we were transferring hatching blastocysts, but we quickly realised that they looked completely different to this one. This blastocyst was actually hatching. Transfer was done and we headed off for our two-week wait.

I was on a lot of post-transfer medications this time, including progesterone support and Pregnyl® boosters. At 13dpt, I started spotting and then my period broke through all the medications. The nurses told me that couldn't happen, but it did! It was another negative cycle for us. The doctor called me and the only advice they had was, 'some women just never fall pregnant'. I couldn't believe the change in attitude. I felt like the doctor had realised I wouldn't be an easy, positive statistic and pushed me to the side.

I was so furious that I went on another rampage to get second opinions, from two other doctors at two different clinics. Neither doctor could believe what had been said to me but they both assured me that I wasn't a lost cause yet. One of the doctors specialised in immune protocols and sent me for more tests. The conclusion was that he wouldn't put me on an immune protocol. I was thinking about moving clinics again but the issue was that we still had seven vials of sperm left. This doctor suggested that I transfer my last embryo and see what happened.

The second doctor did an ultrasound and suggested I try a medication that would clear my uterus of any infection or possible endometriosis, and then transfer my last embryo and see what happened. I decided to try this medication, which was an implant that was put under the skin – a cancer drug that had side effects, such as hot flushes, nausea, headaches and moodiness. I was starting a new job and was assured that not many women get side effects.

Well, I got them all. I started my new job so nauseous that I had hot chips for lunch almost every day for a few weeks and I had intense hot flushes. It was the middle of winter and all of a sudden, I would burn up and get all sweaty. People at my new job must have wondered what the hell was wrong with me. It was awful.

I had the last dose of medication and was ready to start a transfer cycle as soon as my period began… but we waited and waited and waited. 90 days later, I contacted my clinic and told a little lie (as they didn't know I was on this other medication) and said I didn't know why I hadn't got my period yet. It turns out I had a huge cyst on my ovary. I was given a trigger shot and told I would probably get my period in two weeks' time.

I did, and we decided to do a frozen transfer on a natural cycle. It was a strange cycle – there were no injections, no medications, and I didn't know what to do with myself. Transfer happened to fall on a Saturday, which was nice and easy, and it was over with quickly. The embryo looked great and everyone wished us luck. The transfer was also two days before my birthday – I'd always hoped to be pregnant on my birthday and for this cycle, I technically was.

I went to acupuncture, which I'd been doing the whole time but I had a new acupuncturist this time. I walked into the room and she said: 'Congratulations! How are you feeling?'. I looked at her blankly. She continued on with: 'How many weeks are you now?'. I just looked at her and said: 'I'm not pregnant'. She got all flustered and said: 'Oh, I must be thinking of someone else'. At that point, I knew it was my brother's wife, as we have the same surname and went to the same acupuncture clinic. I was so angry and devastated! The first grandchild was meant to be mine, and now it wouldn't be – I felt like my child would always be second. This started off a horrible end to the year.

At first, I thought I wasn't pregnant and the cycle had failed, but just before test day, I started getting slight symptoms. One night, on the way home from work, something kept telling me to go and buy a pregnancy test. Amanda was out that night so I decided to do a test. It came up with a faint positive; I couldn't believe it. I showed Amanda when she got home and she didn't want to know.

I woke up the next morning and tested again – the line was the same colour; I had no idea what to think. It was a Thursday and I headed into the clinic to get my pregnancy test and waited all day for the results. The nurse called me and told me there was HCG in my system but not high enough, so it was either another chemical pregnancy or an ectopic pregnancy. I was shocked but she was unfazed. She told me to come back for a test in two days to check the levels had gone down and hung up. I called Amanda to tell her, by then, we were both pretty numb. That night, we sat at home and cried, we just couldn't believe it was happening again. A couple of hours later, I got a phone call from my brother and he happily announced: 'We are 10 weeks pregnant!'.

We didn't know what to say and neither of us had a great reaction. They asked how we were and I responded with: 'Well, I'm in the middle of a miscarriage'. It was awkward and we finished the phone call. By this time, we were almost three years into TTC and the infertile jealousy and rage I felt towards pregnancy announcements was real and overwhelming – it was almost like I would black out and another personality would take over me.

I went back for another blood test on the Saturday. When the nurse called with my results, the HCG had gone up! They told me it was too low to be a viable pregnancy and to come back in on Monday for another blood test, but my period would probably start over the weekend. On Monday, I had another blood test to check my levels. That day, I also had an initial appointment with another doctor within the same clinic – one of the head doctors of the practice. We were tossing up staying with the same clinic or trying to move our donor sperm to another clinic.

I was armed with a million questions. This was the first time I was seeing a male doctor; I was a little nervous about that but had gotten to the point where I didn't care. The doctor was lovely and answered all my questions before I even asked them. He questioned why I was on such a high dose of medication and told me that sometimes the higher dose can diminish egg quality. He questioned why I'd used ICSI when there was no male factor infertility. He was horrified by the comments made by my previous doctor and he assured me that it wasn't over for me yet. He wanted to watch my natural cycle and do an IUI, so the cycle wasn't completely wasted, and if that didn't work do another round of IVF. The doctor said he would manage my chemical pregnancy. Everything sounded great and we were both really happy with the plan.

As we were walking out, Amanda got a phone call from her brother and went outside to take it. I was paying the bill when I could hear her in the corridor shouting: 'NO, NO, NO!'. The receptionist looked at me and asked if everything was ok, as Amanda ran in with the phone and just said 'I can't', handed me the phone and walked out. I picked up the phone and it was her mum. Amanda's uncle had passed away very unexpectedly.

The rest of the day was a whirlwind. I was cramping, in pain and exhausted, and I had to think quick, get Amanda into a taxi and get her to her brother's house. The nurse called with my results that afternoon and my HCG levels had gone up; I didn't think the day could get any worse. I sat silently, in the middle of a grieving family, knowing this pregnancy wasn't going to last, but starting to feel pregnancy symptoms. That night, I started vomiting for the first time.

My HCG finally went down and my period arrived; it was time to start tracking IUI four. Amanda was a mess so I tried not to worry her with all the details. I did the rough calculations on when the IUI would probably be and it was right around the day of the funeral. The nursing staff knew the situation and were lovely. On the morning of the funeral, I was up early to go and get a blood test, hoping that I wouldn't get the call to say I needed to be back at the clinic that afternoon for the IUI.

Luckily, the lab rushed my results through and the nurse called me to tell me that it wouldn't be that day. IUI day came and my doctor was away – we had his offsider and that was fine. The timing looked perfect. I had a huge dominant follicle, bigger than any of the follicles I'd had before. It was going to be a long two-week wait with those extra five days and not knowing if an egg had fertilised at all.

During the TWW we got more bad news – Amanda's dog wasn't well and we'd known the time was coming to say goodbye but we hadn't thought it would be so soon. Unfortunately, we had to make the decision to say goodbye to her. How many things could go wrong in 2019?!

I knew I wasn't pregnant and once again, my period broke through the medications and came earlier than expected. After 12 attempts at getting pregnant, we were broke. All our hard work and sacrifice on savings had gone nowhere. I desperately wanted to start another IVF cycle in 2019, but not transfer until 2020 for rebate purposes, plus I had three weeks off over Christmas. The doctor was fine with that and decided a long down regulation cycle was the best option for me, with a lower dose of medications and standard IVF as opposed to ICSI.

On Christmas Day 2019, I started injections. Christmas Day was also the first time I saw my brother and sister-in-law in person and everyone had bought the baby presents. It was so tough and I completely broke down after.

This IVF cycle was a bit easier, not having to juggle full-time work and appointments. I was able to relax, eat well and get my body ready for egg collection. I couldn't believe how different this cycle was. My follicles were bigger, my hormone levels were higher. I was usually triggered when my follicles were 16mm and my oestrogen was 5000, but this time, I was triggered when my follicles were over 20mm and my oestrogen was 10,000. Egg collection was a success and 10 eggs were collected. They were going to be fertilised by IVF, with ICSI as a last resort.

I was nervous, but the doctor was so reassuring. The next day, the embryologist called with the fertilisation report: eight eggs fertilised! It was a great result! We were given access to watch our embryos grow and I looked at the pictures obsessively. The day 3 call came from the embryologist and she said that all eight embryos were still developing – it all seemed too good to be true! A couple were a little slower but so far, so good.

Day 5 came and we went in for our transfer. I couldn't believe it when the embryologist came in and told me that all eight embryos were still growing! I wanted to transfer two embryos but the doctor and embryologist talked me out of it for this transfer. The doctor knelt beside me, held my hand and told me this was my time. We transferred a nice looking, hatching blastocyst. Three embryos were also able to be PGS tested. This was turning out to be our best cycle yet. I went to work straight after the transfer, as I couldn't afford to take any more time off.

The next night, Amanda was out and I felt the pulling sensation in my uterus that I'd felt every time I'd fallen pregnant. I thought: 'Surely that's not implantation?!'. I kept that information to myself. A few more days passed and I was convinced that it had failed again. I waited until 13dpt to do my first at-home test. I woke up at 4am, did the test and went back to bed. I wasn't going to bother waiting for the result because I didn't want to see a negative again.

When my alarm went off at 6am, I had to psych myself to get up. I went into the bathroom and stood there, again psyching myself up to look at the test. Eventually, I turned it over and it was positive! I stood

259

there staring at it for ages, not knowing what to do. It was a huge shock and my heart was pounding. I decided I wouldn't tell Amanda yet. The next morning, I did another test and again had to psych myself up because I was convinced it was probably going to be a chemical again and the line would have faded. It hadn't… it was darker! Amanda was meant to be out with work that night so I planned to hold my pee for as long as I could and do another test that night, to possibly showing her when she got home.

She ended up getting sick and came home from work early – my plan was failing already and I didn't think I would be able to hold the news in for another two days, until the beta blood test. I went to the bathroom after dinner and did another test – as soon as I peed on it, the test line started showing up. The line was so dark and so strong, there was no denying that this was looking good. I thought sharing the news would cheer Amanda up, so I called her into the bathroom. She saw I had tests laying out and just started saying: 'No, no, no! I don't want to know; I don't want to see it'. Her reaction was less than desirable and pretty upsetting. I knew it had been a hard road but we needed to celebrate the little wins together.

Friday came and it was blood test day. It was a long wait for the nurse to call, even though she called at 10:30am. I was pregnant! I called Amanda, shaking. It was exciting but also terrifying. I had a big smile on my face all morning. Just after lunch, my bubble was burst when the embryologist called with the PGS testing results: 'I hear you've had some good news this morning! I'm really sorry, but I don't have good news for you'.

Two of the PGS embryos were chromosomally abnormal and were to be discarded, and the third was a chaotic mosaic embryo (which had both normal and abnormal cells). She tried to assure me the results meant nothing in relation to our current pregnancy but when we'd had so many problems, it seemed like this pregnancy was doomed. At first, I started getting pregnancy symptoms and my HCG was rising perfectly. We thought maybe we'd be lucky enough this time, but shortly after, my symptoms started to fade.

At seven weeks, we went for our first ultrasound. We were both so terrified and triggered by the appointment. The night before, Amanda had asked me what my gut feeling was with this pregnancy and I'd told her I thought it was another missed miscarriage. The technician was very understanding and assured us that she would explain what was happening at each step. When the ultrasound started, we could clearly see that this pregnancy looked different. The gestational sac was much bigger and we could both see a flickering heartbeat.

Amanda is a drummer, so it wasn't long before she said to the technician: 'The heartbeat isn't in rhythm'. The technician said it was a bit irregular and baby was measuring a bit small. At this stage with a natural conception, it would be assumed that maybe your dates were wrong, but with IVF there are no mistaking dates. The technician said this can happen and everything could be fine but she suspected I would probably miscarry again – we appreciated her honesty.

We sat in a tiny room, waiting for the doctor's instructions on next steps. While we were waiting, Amanda's phone was going off with messages from work, telling her to jump on a meeting if she could. As we sat there, knowing this pregnancy wasn't going to stick around, Amanda found out she was going to be made redundant. We both looked at each other and laughed – at this point our bad luck was ridiculous; we felt like we couldn't catch a break. The doctor advised me to come back in a week for a follow-up scan but said if I started bleeding or cramping, to get to an emergency department as soon as I could.

A week later, we went in for another scan and my gut told me things weren't right, but this pregnancy wasn't over yet. I was right: baby had grown and the heartbeat had sped up, but it still wasn't normal. We were sent away again, and again told to come back in a week. After the terrible experience I'd had with the D&C at my local public hospital, I enquired with my IVF doctor whether they could do it at their facilities. The receptionist was shocked I was asking but I knew things were not going well and I wanted to be prepared and have everything in place. I pencilled in a date for after my next scan.

We went back to the ultrasound clinic for a third scan, this time with the practice doctor. My eyes locked to the screen and I held my breath. 'I'm sorry, there's no heartbeat' and the screen was quickly switched off. We weren't surprised. We were devastated but it felt like we'd been going through three weeks of grieving at that point. We both knew what to expect and it felt like we were running on autopilot, putting our plan into action. On that day, we knew that was it for my eggs. We couldn't go through all of this again; I would never have a genetic child.

Two days later, in February 2020, we went to our IVF clinic for my D&C. The experience was starkly different. There was no waiting around, I knew all the staff, and they were kind and compassionate to both of us. I went in and woke up to my doctor holding my hand. I was told the procedure had gone well and the pregnancy contents had been sent off for genetic testing. I was given a heat pack, tea and raisin toast. Amanda was always by my side. This time, I was provided with information on what to expect and organisations I could contact for support. So simple, but it made all the difference.

At some point between the last two cycles, the anxiety was too much and I was diagnosed with PTSD. Starting on medication was a hard choice but something I needed to do. It's been one of the better decisions I've made in this journey.

As everyone knows, 2020 went downhill after that. Amanda and I started working from home in March 2020 and throughout the lockdown in Sydney. We didn't know what our next steps were – reciprocal IVF? Find an egg or embryo donor? The plan was still for me to carry a baby if possible. We were going to be working from home for the foreseeable future, so Amanda decided that if there was ever a good time for her to do an egg retrieval, it would be while she could hide away at home.

Our doctor agreed that reciprocal IVF was the best course of action for our next step. The evidence was that my eggs were poor quality, but I had actually fallen pregnant 7 out of 10 times, so using a 'donor embryo' was promising. We started Amanda's first IVF cycle in June 2020 – something that was never in our plan. Our doctor didn't like to do fresh embryo transfers in reciprocal IVF cycles because it was too risky to get both cycles in sync. That was fine with us, as we didn't want to transfer any untested embryos any more – we needed to minimise our risk as much as possible.

Amanda had a really high AMH level so there were fears she would over stimulate easily. After a couple of scans and blood tests, I was pretty concerned that there were only three dominant follicles. The nurse called and said it was time to trigger but this time, I was well versed. There was a possibility that come day 5, we could have only one embryo to transfer. We spoke to the doctor and he agreed that Amanda's medication could be pushed more for a better result, so we cancelled the cycle.

Amanda started another cycle immediately, in the form of a long down regulation cycle. It was definitely an interesting time for both of us, seeing IVF from the other perspective. Amanda realised that the hormonal rage was real and uncontrollable, and I learnt just how hard it was to be patient.

In July 2020, Amanda went in for her first egg retrieval. For someone who hates medical situations, she did so well and I was so proud. Because of Covid restrictions, I wasn't able to be in the procedure room with her but I was there waiting when she woke up. Amanda had 15 eggs retrieved! 24 hours later, we found out that 10 had fertilised. We were given access to the app to watch Amanda's embryos grow and we could immediately tell the difference in quality between my embryos and Amanda's embryos – hers looked so great. By day 3, all 10 embryos were still growing. We were hopeful but didn't want to get too far ahead of ourselves. On day 5, we couldn't believe it – all 10 embryos were still growing! There were two that were a bit behind so they would be taken to day 6. Six embryos were sent off for PGS testing, which was an incredible result.

We watched the time lapse videos of our embryos that night and nicknamed embryo number seven: 'seven costanza'. We'd never seen an embryo quite like it; it was so lively bouncing around the Petri dish. Neither of us wanted to say it, but we knew that number seven was going to be our baby. A couple of weeks later, we got a call from our clinic's genetic counsellor – four embryos were PGS normal and the other two were slightly mosaic. All up, including the two untested embryos, we had eight of Amanda's embryos in the freezer! We couldn't believe it!

Our doctor retired so we had to move to another doctor within our clinic. I knew how I wanted my frozen transfer to be and didn't want to muck around. Our new doctor was very straightforward and agreed. We decided we would cover all bases before transferring any embryos to me. I was sent for a bunch of blood tests and to see a specialist laparoscopic surgeon to rule out endometriosis. The specialist laparoscopic surgeon was appalled by how I'd been treated by the previous doctor who did my laparoscopic surgery and couldn't believe the mess that had been made of my poor naval.

We timed my surgery so I would go into a frozen transfer right after, as the 'clear out' gives you a slightly higher chance of implantation. I'd had a rough 2020, having already had two surgeries on my spine, so my body was not in peak condition. In October 2020, I went in for my laparoscopic surgery – my fifth surgery of the year. All blood tests and the laparoscopic surgery results came back normal once again. I was given the all clear to do our first reciprocal IVF transfer.

In November 2020, we started our cycle. At that point, it had been almost 12 months since I'd taken IVF medications. I felt like a lot was at stake and this would be the decider of my body being able to carry a pregnancy. We had just sold our apartment and it was looking like transfer day was going to be the same day as the removalists were booked in … it was.

On the 9th November 2020, I headed in for a frozen

transfer by myself, while Amanda stayed with the removalists. We both had a renewed sense of hope for this transfer and as we predicted, embryo number seven was the embryo we would be transferring! The embryo looked so great up on the screen before transfer, rolling around and looking very lively again.

I headed off for my 14th two-week wait with only Amanda, myself and my parents knowing about the transfer. Two days later, it was my birthday and I felt that same pulling feeling. I kept it to myself but it felt so magical that I got to feel that sensation on my birthday. On a Sunday morning, at 11dpt, I did my first home pregnancy test. It was positive and quite dark for 11dpt but I couldn't believe it just yet.

On Monday morning (12dpt), the line was darker and I debated whether to tell Amanda yet or not. Mid-morning, we got a call to go into the hospital to say goodbye to our friend, who had been battling cancer – the same good friend who'd introduced Amanda and I years earlier. I sat in the hospital room saying goodbye, knowing I was pregnant – it was such a strange moment of life in full circle. We were both devastated. It was so unfair someone so young was losing their life. It wasn't the day to tell Amanda.

The next day, I went into the clinic for a progesterone check blood test. The nurse called around lunch time and I was armed with a pen in hand to note my progesterone level.

'Congratulations!' she said.

I honestly had no idea what she was talking about.

'Your HCG is 98.7!'

I'd had no idea they were testing my HCG. I couldn't believe it – Amanda's embryo had worked! I was pregnant. I thought about elaborate ways to tell Amanda but in the end, I went into the room where she was working, with the camera rolling.

'Guess what?!'

She looked at me blankly.

'It worked!'

Still nothing.

'Your embryo… it worked!'

She dropped her head in her hands and cried. I was finally able to surprise her.

As I write this, I am 20 weeks pregnant and our little rainbow baby is kicking away. The first weeks of pregnancy were the longest weeks of my life, filled with anxiety. We have chosen to have our care through a private obstetrician and that has been the best decision for us. My OB has been great and really understanding of my anxiety and PTSD. I've been referred to a perinatal psychologist and it's made such a difference to have a team around me for support every step of the way.

Around 17 weeks, I started feeling flutters, which was so reassuring, and by 19 weeks, Amanda felt her first kick. Our recent 20-week scan went well and my bump has well and truly popped now.

We feel so incredibly grateful to be pregnant but we are still nervous and not quite there yet. Making it halfway through pregnancy is such an achievement and after everything we've been through, all the years of heartache, it still doesn't seem real. In July 2021, we will be bringing home our rainbow baby. A little boy who will be loved unconditionally. Our lucky embryo number seven.

If you are going through infertility or loss, I see you, I hear you, I am you. You will get through this – you are much stronger than you know.

If you're a family member or a friend who knows someone who is going through infertility or loss, my advice to you is just to be there to listen and support. Unfortunately, no amount of 'it happened for a reason' or 'just relax' is going to change the situation and make us feel any better, but just being there to listen when we need to talk may help a little.

Connect with me on Instagram:
@mummyplusmumma

Chosen charity

Our charity is Pink Elephants:
www.pinkelephants.org.au

Founded in Sydney, they provide resources, information and peer-support to anyone impacted by early pregnancy loss.

Steph and Karl

After five years of TTC and three rounds of
medication, they conceived naturally and had a baby
boy in November 2020. Their journey talks about their
experience with secondary infertility, an early
miscarriage, and the impact this had on a newly
married couple.

Steph

A little introduction to me: My name is Steph, I'm
35 years old and I live in Wolverhampton, West
Midlands. I am a Registered Adult Nurse and have been
a nurse for five years. I started working in health care
when I was 18 years old and after many happy years, I
knew it was time to set myself a challenge and achieve
my nursing degree. I currently work in palliative care
nursing and although some days it can be the hardest
job in the world, it's definitely the most rewarding.
Apart from becoming a qualified nurse, my biggest
accomplishment has always been becoming a mom.

In September 2005, I gave birth to my beautiful,
healthy, baby boy Luke. From the moment he was in
my arms, I knew how much I loved and adored him.
Although only 20 years old, being a mom came
naturally. I felt ready for motherhood. I had a lot of
support from my family and Luke's father's family
over the years. However, my relationship with Luke's
father ended when Luke was two years old. A few years
later, in 2011, I met Karl unexpectedly through social
media. Nine years later, we are married and now a
family of four. We got married in August 2015 and
what a year it was. We both turned 30 years old, got
married and bought a house. That's when the next part
of our journey started.

Our story starts like most couples – married, new
house, new baby… well, that's how we'd hoped it

would be. Myself and Karl couldn't wait to be parents. Although already a parent, I couldn't wait to have another child. A few months after we married, we decided it was time to start trying for a baby. I had my intrauterine device removed and would let nature take its course. As easy as getting pregnant was the first time, I never imagined it would be any different this time.

After a year of trying to conceive (TTC), with no signs of a pregnancy, we decided it was time to see a doctor. After visiting the GP, we were told to continue trying, and the doctor informed us that it can take couples one or two years to conceive. I felt like this was an attempt to try and reassure us that 12 months wasn't too long to be trying, while feeling like the appointment was a waste of time. We continued again, now reaching 18 months of TTC. I was starting to worry about why this wasn't happening for us. I began doubting myself, that maybe there was something wrong with me. Surely there couldn't be though – I already had a child so I'd conceived naturally once before. Although, I knew that being much older this time, my fertility would start declining.

We headed back to the GP, wanting to know why it still wasn't happening for us. This time, she recommended we have some blood tests done and for Karl to do a sperm sample for analysis. Each month, discovering we had been unsuccessful was becoming more and more frustrating. We couldn't figure out where we were going wrong. With our blood tests done and Karl's sperm sample sent, it was a case of waiting to see what the results showed.

Over the coming months, I downloaded a fertility app to log my menstrual cycle and track my ovulation to work out the timing for the next month, but I seemed to be inconsistent with periods. With only a few days each cycle to conceive, I was sure we were trying at the wrong time. I found myself in an endless cycle of tracking and planning my ovulation days. After not feeling reassured with the app, I began using the Clearblue® digital ovulation tests for more accuracy. These tests slowly started to control each month – I would wait to see that smiley, flashing face on the test before we would try to conceive. Spontaneous and passionate sex with my husband wasn't the plan any more, it was more the process of trying to conceive; turning sex into a military operation. We would only try when the test said I was ovulating, so we focused on that small window of time. Some months became a 'wasted' month when we had missed our ovulation window for one reason or the other. Those months just became no pressure months, with no symptom checking or worrying.

In December 2017, I wasn't feeling great and neither was my son, so I just assumed we both weren't well. After a chat with my sister-in-law, telling her how I felt, she encouraged me to take a pregnancy test. I was only a couple of days late but with my irregular periods, this was nothing new. We never imagined the outcome to be anything other than what we had experienced so many times before when taking pregnancy tests. This time was different though, it was positive. We were pregnant! That one little word hit us like a ton of bricks. We honestly did not expect to see a positive pregnancy test. We made an appointment to see our GP and waited excitedly to see the new year in.

A few days later, I started to have a bleed – nothing major, but enough to have me worried. After visiting our local walk-in centre and being checked over, along with a confirmed pregnancy test, I was told I was too early to be seen at the EPAU. From my calculated dates, I would've only been around five weeks pregnant at the time and the bleeding could have been what was called implantation bleeding. I had never heard of this before, so after a quick Google, we found out it was actually quite common in early pregnancy and seemed to be the same as what I was experiencing.

However, over the next couple of days, the bleeding began to increase and I was starting to get concerned. One evening, after ringing NHS 111 for advice, I was advised to visit an out of hours GP. The doctor we saw that night was blunt and unsympathetic to our situation. She carried out a pregnancy test from my urine sample – it was negative! She told us we were not pregnant and sent us home. Before I had even got outside and reached the car, I was in floods of tears. This was the first positive pregnancy test we'd had through the whole time TTC, I didn't want to believe we weren't pregnant that quickly.

Out of interest the next morning, I did another home pregnancy test – it was positive. Two clear blue lines. We were so confused. How could it be positive when the day before we were told it was negative? I turned to Google again and looked up anything from false negative/positive pregnancy tests, types of pregnancy tests and the best time to take a test. I needed answers. I went to work as normal that week but I knew something was wrong – the bleeding had increased and I was having awful cramping pains. On the 2nd January, we went back to see our GP, who confirmed what we already expected – our pregnancy test was negative and with the symptoms from the previous days, it was explained that this was an early miscarriage. We were heartbroken. In only that short space of time, it gave us hope that we could conceive, that I wasn't broken or Karl wasn't the reason for us not getting pregnant. As early as it may have been to not be pregnant any more, the loss hurt just as much.

We returned back to the GP, after receiving a phone call to discuss our test results. The results had shown that Karl's sperm sample was good, however my blood test had highlighted an abnormal level with one of my hormones. With our time period of trying to conceive and other contributing factors, we were diagnosed with secondary infertility. She explained to us that this was the inability to conceive or carry a baby to full term after successfully becoming pregnant at least once before. Although secondary infertility is similar to other types of infertility and shares many of the same signs, factors like age, health, obesity, and stress can be the cause. I had never heard of secondary infertility or knew of anyone who was having the same difficulties as myself to be able to relate too. This was all new to us. Even going through the rest of our journey, the term 'secondary infertility' wasn't something I came across from other women when I would explain why I wasn't getting pregnant. We were referred to a Gynaecology consultant at our local hospital for further tests and treatment.

We booked a holiday in May 2018 to Jamaica, to just enjoy being the family we already were. We were also hoping the holiday would help us unwind and rekindle some of the passion in our marriage. Infertility can bring a range of challenging emotions, such as sadness, hopelessness, confusion, frustration, and even guilt. I think over the years, I had experienced them all but I was not prepared for the guilt I felt as a parent. I felt guilty that I already had a child and all my attention over the last year had been so focused on wanting another baby that I wasn't enjoying enough time with the one I had.

Our first meeting with our consultant went well. He was friendly and informative, and he instantly made us feel relaxed. My blood test results showed I had low progesterone levels, causing irregular or absent menstrual cycles. I wasn't aware that adequate progesterone levels were crucial in order to maintain pregnancy; and that low luteal phase progesterone levels were also associated with an increased risk of implantation failure and can commonly lead to early miscarriage. This explained a lot!

Our consultant explained our options going forward, in the hope they would help us conceive before having to think about IVF treatment. I knew in the back of my mind this was always going to be one of our options but I wanted to try anything that could potentially help us conceive first. After having my uterus examined to rule out any potential causes, we were prescribed a six-month course of an oral fertility medication, called Clomid®, to start.

In June 2018, I was back at the hospital for my hysteroscopy. This was just a 30-minute procedure in which a hysteroscope is inserted through the cervix into the uterus to give a clear view of the opening of the fallopian tubes – a procedure that is used to look at the cervix and uterus for anything abnormal. Although not painful, it was uncomfortable and I felt self-conscious. The results had shown my tubes were clear but I had a polyp that needed to be removed. This was just the next step of trying to rule out anything that could be adding to us not getting pregnant, but this also meant we could start the medication our consultant had prescribed.

Apprehensive about taking Clomid®, I wanted to know more about it. I wanted to be sure it was safe to take and what the possible outcome this medication had when taken for infertility complications like mine. I found that Clomid® is considered to be the 'first-line' fertility medication, used to treat a range of infertility factors but usually those related to irregular ovulation. I was hoping this would be the answer to us getting pregnant, as it had a good success rate. As instructed, I started my cycle of Clomid® on the second day of my menstrual cycle, for the next five days. In order to see if I had ovulated and the medication was working, I needed to have a blood test performed on day 21 of my menstrual cycle, to measure my progesterone levels. Finally, some good news – my blood test results from August had shown that my serum progesterone levels had increased to 44.3nmol/l. This was definite evidence I was ovulating and very reassuring. The letter from my consultant made me smile. He had written to inform us of our results and to advise us to arrange a further appointment if unsuccessful after the six months, but it was the way he'd ended the letter with a little note that caused the smile – he said, 'Continue to wine and dine each other on a regular basis'.

Nothing can prepare you for the battle against infertility. We had spent month after month, year after year, revolving our life around having a baby. The strain it puts on your marriage is a different type of strain. You're together on a journey that only you as a couple can understand; as much as you try to explain to your loved ones, they never truly understand. You're fighting together for something you both want so badly, that in the end you start to fight against each other. I had times when I thought our marriage wouldn't survive. Times I thought I couldn't give my husband the one thing he was desperate for. Times I said to him to go be with someone else. We were exhausted!

Unsuccessful with our course of Clomid®, we were

back meeting our Gynaecology consultant in January 2019. Again, we discussed our options. We were prescribed a three-month course of Letrozole – another oral hormone fertility medication. Originally created to treat breast cancer, Letrozole also helps induce ovulation. It works by increasing your chances of releasing more than one egg, which, in turn, improves your odds of getting pregnant. Again, I was apprehensive about taking another hormone medication. Although I didn't get many side effects from Clomid®, other than headaches, Letrozole made me feel ill. I felt tired, my mood swings were up and down and I felt nauseous all the time. I couldn't wait to finish taking them.

By April 2019 I was exhausted. I had given up. I didn't want to take any more medication or have any more tests. Me and Karl were arguing more and more. With each pregnancy announcement from friends or family it became harder and harder. It wasn't a case of not being happy for them, it was just so disheartening that it wasn't us. I needed some time to feel like myself again. I decided to go away for a week and spend some time with Luke and my best friend. In a positive way, the break from Karl was needed for both of us.

Three months passed by and with every 'just relax, it will happen' or 'everything happens for a reason' comment, I was starting to become more upset and angry. What if it didn't happen for us? We'd had the conversation about IVF but along with the stress of TTC, also came the stress of having to pay for IVF treatment if this was our only option. Due to me already having a child from my previous relationship, NHS funding is not normally available. There are exceptions where the child is not the biological child of both partners, but this would depend on the fertility policy of the local Clinical Commissioning Group (CCG). Our consultant had made us aware from our previous appointment that we would not be entitled to funding and would have to pay privately if we did consider this in the future.

We went back to see our Gynaecology consultant again for the third time. We'd discussed as a couple that we didn't want any more medication. We couldn't take trying like that any longer and we just wanted a referral for IVF. With that in mind, our consultant discussed this with us and agreed. He suggested in the meantime, while we wait, to try another three-month course of Letrozole, along with another oral medication called Provera®. Provera® (Medroxyprogesterone) is given to replace the progesterone hormone when your body isn't making enough of it. As with both the previous medications, my day 21 blood tests had indicated I was ovulating, as my levels had increased with both courses.

I explained I wasn't keen on taking any more medication but with how I was already feeling, I thought I had nothing to lose by trying. How wrong I was. I felt even worse taking Provera®. My body ached, I felt bloated and was having awful headaches. I couldn't take any more of feeling like this, so after discussing with Karl, we agreed to stop the medication and see the rest of the year out. Another new year came and we felt relaxed going into 2020, knowing there would be no more medication and we could look to start IVF.

Although I didn't plan to continue taking Provera® any longer – due to the nature of the medication it should not be taken when pregnant. As advised by our consultant, in the event of becoming pregnant I would need to stop taking Provera® and commence using progesterone pessaries, called Cyclogest®. These were vaginal pessaries containing progesterone, which are normally prescribed to support early pregnancy in women who've had IVF treatment. The progesterone acts on the womb lining and causes it to thicken in preparation for a fertilised egg to implant. This increases the chance of a successful pregnancy.

I had finished taking Provera® on day 28 of my menstrual cycle, as this was normally a typical cycle length for me. On what should've been the first day of my period, I was advised to take a pregnancy test in order to know if to continue with Provera® or stop. I didn't plan to continue with any of the medication, so didn't see the point in taking another pregnancy test for it to just be negative. I was adamant that it couldn't be positive as previous medications hadn't worked for us, so why would this one be any different? I went out and bought a pregnancy test anyway to put Karl's mind at ease and I figured even if it was negative, at least we would know for sure. Again, like so many times before, we didn't expect anything less than those two heart breaking words 'not pregnant'.

This time it was positive! I checked and checked the pregnancy test to make sure the pregnant sign didn't disappear. I was in shock. Although I didn't want to tell Karl over the phone as he was at work, I couldn't wait for him to get home. Over the next couple of days, I lost track of how many different pregnancy tests I took, just to make sure it was real. With each blue line or positive word came excitement and fear. I made an appointment with the midwife and waited anxiously.

Ten days later, after experiencing lower abdominal pain and heavy bleeding, we attended A&E. All the signs and fears from our last miscarriage came rushing back, and we were terrified it was happening again.

After another positive pregnancy test and no signs of infection, we were none the wiser to what was going on. The doctor we saw that night was so lovely. She reassured us this could be normal at this point but could not confirm if we were still pregnant or if we were in the early stage of miscarriage. It was too early to be seen at the EPAU so we were sent home on bed rest and advised to continue the pessaries until confirmed not pregnant. After our visit to A&E, we were referred to the EPAU at our local hospital for an ultrasound scan. Myself and Karl had convinced ourselves we had miscarried again and went to the appointment expecting to hear those words.

The consultant informed us the ultrasound findings showed an abnormal gestational sac, representative of an early miscarriage. I had some blood tests taken and went home to break the news to the few family members who knew we were pregnant. The next day, after receiving a phone call to say my HCG levels were high, we headed back to the hospital for a rescan to confirm the ultrasound findings. We were met by a consultant who wanted to rule out an ectopic or multiple pregnancy. This time, the ultrasound showed a normal gestational sac, with a tiny flicker of a heartbeat. We were pregnant after all!

All happy tears aside, the good news came with some not so good news. There was a large haematoma adjacent to the sac, which was causing the bleeding. We left with instructions to go back for a rescan two weeks later. We were worried about telling family members who knew we were pregnant that we hadn't miscarried – we were still pregnant but not to get too excited. The consultant had explained that the haematoma could result in pregnancy loss. Subchorionic hematoma's can increase the risk of an array of pregnancy complications, including miscarriage, preterm labour and placental abruption. Most subchorionic bleeds resolve on their own, and lead to perfectly healthy pregnancies. We just had to pray this was the case for us.

My anxiety during those two weeks was so bad. I would always try to be positive but also prepare myself for the worst-case scenario and I would just swing between the two, counting down the days until the next scan. As advised, I had taken some time off work to avoid strenuous activity and rest. After the longest two weeks, we were back at the hospital. Sat in the waiting room with my husband, who was being positive for the both of us, I was sure it was going to be bad news. Thankfully, it wasn't – we were still pregnant. The haematoma was still there but had reduced slightly in size. I was advised to continue to rest and come back in four weeks' time.

On 22nd April, we were back for our 12-week scan. The bleeding had reduced significantly. I was starting to feel pregnant now – nausea was becoming daily and I had gone off food and drinks I enjoyed. I felt more positive this time. Everything looked good on the scan. There was our baby, being mischievous and not keeping still. No haematoma to be seen, so we were given the all clear. Our baby had grown so much. I lay on the hospital bed in floods of happy and relieved tears. I was so overwhelmingly in love with our baby already.

The weeks rolled on and at 16 weeks we decided to pay for a private gender scan, as we were not only impatient to find out the sex of our baby, but also so my husband could be present for the scan. Who would've thought after waiting all those years to conceive, I would now be pregnant in a pandemic! Karl wasn't allowed to attend the scans at the hospital so this was the only way he could experience the joy of seeing our baby together. We were expecting a boy!

Growing closer and closer to our due date, we became more excited and impatient. Our due date arrived and passed by – there were no signs of our baby making an arrival anytime soon. Eleven days overdue, I was taken into hospital to be induced. After the craziest pregnancy, all I wanted was a natural birth. My plans for a water birth were no longer allowed due to being induced but I knew I wanted to do it as naturally as possible. I should have known it was never going to be that simple. On the 1st November, I was rushed to theatre for an assisted birth after a traumatic labour. At 19:50 our baby boy, Finley, made his entrance into the world.

Having our tiny, beautiful baby here now, in our arms, has made the last five years and everything we've been through worth it. Not that the journey to get where we are now doesn't matter anymore, because it absolutely does. It made us who we are as parents, as a couple, and as a completed family of four.

Connect with me on Instagram:
@mummy_and_finley

Chosen charity

Our charity is one that is very close to us as a family, The Bumpy Foundation:
www.facebook.com/thebumpyfoundation

They raise money to help families who are currently coping with the loss of a baby in pregnancy or childbirth.

Aisha and Billahl

Childfree after infertility

This couple spent 10 years trying to conceive –
a late diagnosis of stage IV endometriosis revealed
the primary cause of Aisha's infertility. Over 11
unsuccessful IVF attempts and many miscarriages
later, they decided to embrace their childfree-after-
infertility life. With real courage and determination,
they eventually got to a place of healing and
acceptance. They share their infertility journey in the
hope that it will inspire others. Aisha and Billahl are
living proof that it is possible to live a happy life
beyond being a parent, even if it's not the one
you planned.

Introducing myself

I'm Aisha. I live in North London with my wonderful husband, Billahl, and our cat, Peaches, the most adorable cream, British shorthair. Billahl and I married in 2005 and in 2009, we started our long journey towards parenthood. The whole of my thirties was consumed by infertility and trying to conceive – I underwent surgery for endometriosis, numerous rounds of IVF and multiple miscarriages. I eventually decided to give infertility the middle finger and embrace a childfree-after-infertility life.

Something I realised while going through my infertility experience was that, while there is a lot more awareness being created for those who have been diagnosed with infertility, miscarriage and neonatal loss, there's nothing much for those of us who leave the process childless.

When I eventually stopped trying to conceive, I started to really think about what I wanted from life. In early 2020, I left my job working at a Trust Fund company and started mindbodyrevival_coach. It's something I'm incredibly proud of. My main aim when starting my coaching practice was to support my clients' thinking. This includes anyone from the infertility community to those working in the business world. I absolutely love working with people, whatever stage of their infertility journey, and particularly those who are childfree after infertility, like me. The work I do is such a privilege, and it has been wonderful to see the transformation in all of my clients – it has also been an important part of my own healing.

Given my history and experience, I have also become an endometriosis, miscarriage and childfree advocate – topics that are all close to my heart. In this chapter, I'll be covering all three topics.

My infertility journey

My fertility journey started almost 11 years ago, long before the creation of fertility-related Instagram or Facebook accounts that can now be used as a source of information, support and community. It was a very lonely time.

Unbeknown to me, the issues at the root of my infertility started a long time before I'd even thought about having a child, when I was 15 years old. I started experiencing dreadful pain during menstruation – pain which grew worse as the years went on. My mum was extremely concerned and took me to see a doctor. It may come as no surprise, given the history of medical gaslighting when it comes to women's pain, but the agony I was experiencing was dismissed as 'bad periods'. Regrettably, research suggests that things haven't changed much when it comes to medical gaslighting, especially with illnesses such as endometriosis and PCOS.

In between school and university, I saw several consultants. Each one saying the same thing: 'there's nothing wrong with you'. One doctor even suggested that I see a psychologist because she believed that the pain was psychological – this makes me chuckle now, bearing in mind the severity of the symptoms that I was displaying. At the time, I felt completely helpless and hopeless.

The pain I was experiencing worsened in my late teens and early twenties. I'll describe an unfortunate incident when I visited my GP 16 years ago, when my pain was at its peak – a memory that remains vivid all these years later. I was studying for a Master's degree and my exams were looming. I remember not being able to revise much because the pain in my stomach was so intense that it left me confined to my bed. At that time in my life, excruciating pain was a daily occurrence that became the norm, intensifying during menstruation. I was forced to remain bedbound for 14 days each month – I felt as though I couldn't carry on living with the excruciating pain.

I sat down and explained my symptoms: nausea, extreme fatigue, intolerable pain and excessive bleeding. After a while, I couldn't speak because I was crying so much – I was so upset that I was unable to revise for my exams due to the pain. The doctor looked at me, unresponsive, and proceeded to hand me a tissue. Other than that, he didn't convey much empathy towards me or appear to know what to do about the problem. Apart from being prescribed the oral contraceptive pill and low-dose painkillers (which I had to ask for), I was left to get on with it. From that moment, I realised that I wouldn't be getting the help I desperately needed and deserved. It was clear that no one believed the extent of the pain that I was coping with, each and every day.

A few years later, my husband and I decided we wanted to try for a baby. Although most people are surprised when it doesn't happen immediately, I wasn't – it was a fear I'd had for years. My history of ill health and painful intercourse were all signs that were ignored by medical professionals, but not by me. We tried naturally for two years – nothing happened. Eventually, my GP sent me for blood tests. Two weeks later, I was relieved to hear the results were all normal, and we were told to continue trying to conceive naturally. A year later – still nothing. I went back to the GP, who discovered that the blood test results I'd received the previous year were in fact abnormal – I was devastated.

A late endometriosis diagnosis

My cousin was furious about the treatment I'd received from doctors over the years – enough was enough. She believed I might be suffering with the same condition she had: endometriosis – a condition that wasn't on the radar of most medical professionals. She told me to advocate for myself and self-refer at a hospital outside my borough through my GP. A hospital that specialised in fertility. Six months later, after a 20-minute appointment with a consultant, I was told that I displayed many symptoms associated with endometriosis and that I would need a laparoscopy. I will never forget that moment – the first time that I felt understood and believed.

For those who may not know, endometriosis is a condition where tissue, similar to the lining of the womb, grows in various locations throughout the body. My laparoscopy showed the presence of bilateral endometrioses on both ovaries and on the bowel (my ovaries and bowel were adherent to the uterus) and two endometriomas (chocolate cysts). During the surgery, my ovaries were freed so they were no longer sticking together and the endometriomas were drained. Unfortunately, it was only possible to partially free my bowel. I also had a deep endometriotic nodule which was impossible to remove without having my bowel prepped first.

I felt completely overwhelmed with the information I received after my surgery. What did it mean? Would I be able to have a baby? Was this condition curable? What were my next steps? I remember being in a lot of pain after surgery. My emotions were bitter-sweet – I was happy to finally receive a diagnosis and know that someone 'actually' believed me. Equally, I was sad that it had taken over 15 years to get to this point. I felt as though my diagnosis gave me something to blame and I could now make sense of the struggle.

Moving forward with Assisted Reproductive Technology - IVF

After my laparoscopy, the doctors unanimously agreed that if I pursued IVF, my chances of a successful pregnancy would be much greater than trying naturally. Six months before I started fertility treatment, I received hormones to downregulate my ovaries. I started monthly Zoladex® injections. Zoladex® is believed to reduce endometrial lesions and thin the endometrium – this is why many people with endometriosis have these injections before beginning fertility treatment. Having endometriosis makes IVF more complicated, and taking the injections is believed to reduce inflammation, and may improve IVF success rates for some individuals. Once the six months were completed, I was finally able to start my first IVF cycle through the NHS. It was extremely nerve-racking. I didn't really know what I was doing and I didn't understand many of the protocols. What made it worse was the unfriendly reception staff at the clinic.

Even though my first egg collection was almost 11 years ago now, I remember it vividly because I was so anxious. Fortunately, the egg collection was successful and five eggs were retrieved – I was extremely pleased with this number, considering I also had low AMH. In total, four embryos developed, two were transferred on day 3, one was frozen, and the fourth was discarded. I had no sleep the night before the transfer because I was extremely scared and nervous. The transfer was excruciatingly painful due to the endometriosis that was still present in my bowel – the prerequisite to also have a full bladder during the procedure didn't help either.

A few days post transfer, I knew my treatment hadn't worked – I started bleeding. The bleeding got progressively heavier as the week went on. It was all over. Devastated, the HCG test confirmed what I already knew – I was not pregnant. The frozen embryo transfer that I had a few months later ended the same way – a big, fat, negative. I was only offered two free cycles on the NHS, including the FET. Going forward, if my husband and I wanted to pursue further treatment, it would have to be privately funded.

IVF is expensive for anyone who is self-funding and saving for treatment involves huge sacrifice. IVF was very financially draining on us as a couple, especially because of how many rounds we had. As I rarely had any frozen embryos, each time a cycle would fail, I needed to repeat the entire process. I would also have to have more Zoladex® injections between cycles because of the endometriosis. In total, I had approximately eleven IVF cycles and one IUI.

In between – the difficult emotions

I went through many emotions during my infertility journey, and I personally believe they deserved more acknowledgement and attention than they received. Yes, the physical side of infertility was soul destroying but, quite frankly, the emotional impact was far worse, in my opinion. Holding on to hope and fear in equal measure, day after day for ten years, has an impact on even the toughest individual.

The complex emotions that are a consequence of infertility are extremely under acknowledged. I found it hard to share my voice during those years because my feelings were often misunderstood. Acknowledgement and empathy were hugely lacking – my story would usually evoke pity instead of recognition.

The years spent trying to conceive were the most difficult of my adult life. I wasn't given the space I desperately yearned for in society to express my grief and heartache. Often, those who hadn't a clue about infertility would respond with comments such as, 'just relax', 'maybe it's not meant to be', or 'it's God's will'. Given the gravity of the situation, this was extremely hurtful. These responses downplayed how challenging the struggles of infertility were, and they contributed to even greater anguish, upset and isolation on my part.

Nearly every time I verbalised my suffering, all I wanted to hear were the words; 'I'm so sorry for your horrible situation'. I wanted people to sit with me in the ache and listen. I wanted people to listen without offering unsolicited advice – advice that often left me feeling even more shame, sadness and certainty that I was overreacting. I felt there was little compassion towards the pain my husband and I were experiencing. Those who proclaimed that we shouldn't 'get annoyed' over our situation had clearly never had to deal with infertility for a single day in their lives. How privileged these comments were, being able to distance themselves from anything that could compromise their sunny outlook. *Rolls eyes*.

From my husband's point of view, loneliness due to infertility was something he felt very deeply. He believed that others who hadn't experienced infertility couldn't comprehend the extent of its impact – they had no idea about how severely infertility affects physical and mental health, relationships and finances. Many couldn't see the loneliness he experienced because he was good at hiding it. He didn't feel as though he could talk about it, partly because of the above, and also because in the culture he belongs to, men 'just don't talk about these things'.

Billahl talks about infertility:

I'm a happy-go-lucky guy – this is my personality; I don't know any other way to be. When I'm reminded about the past, I get upset, which is why I don't like talking about what happened. When I do, the grief resurfaces. No one understands the grief and anxiety that comes with seeing your wife enduring round after round of egg collections. Each stage of the process caused grief when it didn't work – there were many milestones we had to reach just to be able to get to the next hurdle, and even after that, there were many more. It can severely affect your mental health. The waiting, oh the pain of waiting – even positive news caused so much anxiety because we were always expecting something to go wrong. In our case, it usually did.

Talking about this experience today, all these years later, left my husband hugely emotional.

My first miscarriage

I cried a great deal during the years when I was trying to conceive. Some days, I couldn't communicate how unhappy I was to my husband, for fear of upsetting him. I was fortunate enough to be able to count on my cousin for support. My cousin lost her son at 26 weeks, a few years prior to my infertility diagnosis. Although she wasn't infertile, it didn't matter – our losses united us, and she proved to be a huge source of comfort during my darkest moments. Many times, she'd come over to my house, and on occasion at absurd hours, to sit with me in the ache when I felt I wasn't coping.

Of all the pregnancy announcements made, the most difficult one to digest was when my mum revealed my sister was expecting. My family were in Saudi Arabia when they shared the news with me via phone. I remember crying for days after hearing the news. I was happy they were away so they couldn't see the state I was in. Of course, I was tremendously happy for my sister, but in that moment, I felt extremely sad for myself.

The next six months represented a funny turn of events. I had my first, positive pregnancy test, on my fourth round of IVF I believe (it's hard to keep track because I have undergone so many). The whole experience was strange. Around seven days post transfer, I started bleeding. There was a lot of blood, so I assumed it was yet another IVF fail. The same week my mum took me shopping to cheer me up. On the morning of the same day, I'd nipped over to Harley

Street to have an HCG test, which I was certain would be negative. My phone rangx whilst I was driving home from the day out. To my astonishment, the result was positive. I was pregnant. No way! How? My husband was over the moon and my family were so happy that my sister and I were pregnant simultaneously. It was a lovely moment my sister and I shared together.

Unfortunately, the joy was short-lived. The bleeding continued for a further few weeks and with it came unbearable, continuous cramping in my stomach and lower back. The pain worsened by the day, and the blood became more intense each time I'd visit the toilet. Oddly, each time I went for a beta test, the numbers increased. I couldn't take any medication for the pain, just in case, and the regular blood tests revealed that I was becoming 'more pregnant', even though all the physical signs suggested otherwise. Approximately six weeks later, an early transvaginal scan revealed that the pregnancy wasn't progressing as expected. A day later, the symptoms of miscarriage came in full force. The pain was excruciating. Heartbreakingly, we had lost our baby.

The next eight years looked very similar – more rounds of egg collections, failed transfers and miscarriages. I also had further surgery and treatment for endometriosis between IVF cycles. This involved more Zoladex® injections and keyhole surgery to drain endometriomas and separate my ovaries – once again, they had become attached to each other. I was becoming tired, and so were my ovaries. Subsequently, I had two more unsuccessful pregnancies: after IVF, I miscarried twins in the second trimester, and a few years later, I had an early miscarriage after an IUI. Nothing seemed to be working for us as a couple. We'd certainly seen IVF success for many other couples over the years, some even having a third round of successful IVF. It was so deflating that we continued to have IVF fails.

With all the heartbreak we endured, the road was becoming increasingly difficult to travel. At this point, we were running out of options and decided to go down the PGS testing route. This came at a huge financial cost but, thinking this may finally be the path to parenthood, we proceeded. After two rounds of egg collections we only had one viable embryo. I had the transfer but, after the long, dreaded two-week wait, we finally received the news: not pregnant! We were at a loss. Our consultant said we were just unlucky this time round and after lengthy discussions, we decided to bank more eggs and have the embryos PGS tested. This would mean another two rounds of egg collections in order to collect enough eggs. It was a lot to consider.

At that point, I wasn't worried about our chances of success. My eggs had consistently been of good quality and the resulting embryos often reached day 5 (blastocyst). After a few months' rest, my husband and I were ready to face the next round of IVF. Tragically, I received news that none of my eggs passed the stress test when thawing. Neither I, my husband, nor the clinical team could believe the outcome considering my history. I was devastated, not to mention deflated, angry, upset and confused. For the first time in my trying to conceive journey, it all proved too much, and I didn't leave my bed for four days. I couldn't eat, I just lay there, sleeping and weeping, wondering why we just couldn't get pregnant. It was at this point that we knew our journey to parenthood was over – the grief and loss were overwhelmingly difficult. Together, we decided that we couldn't cope with more disappointments.

The constant disappointments, along with the intensity of the hormones I had to take for each IVF cycle, contributed to the bad mental health I endured for years. They were the main factors, and good enough reasons, to quit my path to parenthood.

The transition to becoming childfree was a difficult one, but with patience, therapy, faith, healing and lots of support from the best family and friends a couple could ask for, we were able to get through the ache and embrace our childfree-after-infertility life.

Becoming childfree after infertility

My path to healing

Healing is often described as, 'an act of love towards ourselves and others'. Letting go of what was no longer serving me was an act of love towards myself. This meant letting go of trying to conceive, becoming a mother, and being a parent with my husband – all incredibly difficult things to shake. The transition was even more painful than the thought of change. For 10 years, 'I was infertility' – it was my identity. Weekly appointments at the clinic, blood tests and regular procedures were all I knew. I wondered what I'd identify as when this stopped. Saying goodbye to a life I'd been used to felt like a huge loss.

With therapy and lots of self-help, I was eventually able to make it through the sadness and embrace my childfree-after-infertility life. I let go of the idea that my life should look a certain way, and that a childfree life is an empty life – a message often reinforced in the pronatalist society we live in. Through my healing, and as the years have progressed, I have created a life that I absolutely love. It has allowed me to focus on what makes me happiest.

Grief and gratitude can coexist. I have felt sad because of the things I don't have, and at the same time, I have been very grateful for what I do have. I am incredibly grateful to have a husband I adore, family and friends who are beyond amazing, and a cheeky moggy who soothes me on the days when I have an endometriosis flare-up. I'm also thankful I have an amazing job where I get to empower those who are on a similar path to my own. I'm not suggesting I don't encounter problems in life, because everyone does. What it does mean, is that IVF and infertility are no longer the biggest difficulties taking up space in our lives.

The use of toxic language

Many of us who are childfree after infertility feel some of the language used in the wider infertility community needs to be addressed because it reinforces toxic positivity. 'Never give up' is a phrase I see on a lot of social media platforms – as if having a baby is the ONLY acceptable outcome when you're infertile. These words can be a dangerous way of ignoring someone's lived reality and alludes to the fact that at some point, if you try hard enough, you will definitely have a baby. The problem with infertility is that the outcome isn't determined by the effort you put in.

Phrases like this create a sense of false hope and add extra layers of burden, such as guilt and shame when a person wants to walk away from trying to conceive. Saying 'never give up' to someone who is infertile does more harm than good, I believe. It's like throwing shade on the grief of those who have left the process childfree after infertility, reinforcing the fallacy that 'we gave up' – we didn't. Quitting is not shameful. 'Never give up' is the reason why many people stay in bad relationships or carry on in a job they hate – because quitting is synonymous with failure. I think the saying should be rephrased: 'Give up when you're ready'. In many infertility cases, sometimes it is too difficult, too painful or too late to continue trying.

I wish there had been a childless-not-by-choice community 11 years ago – maybe I wouldn't have felt compelled to keep trying and not 'give up'. Perhaps, if I had a community saying it's okay to 'quit', I'd have managed my expectations better and not put myself through so many rounds of IVF. Maybe I would have been more inclined to accept my reality – a reality that severe endometriosis would greatly decrease my chances of having a baby.

When I decided to embrace my childfree-after-infertility life, I wasn't giving up, I was letting go of the pain, disappointment, upset and misery that had consumed my life for so long. It meant I valued my marriage, relationships, physical and mental health, and my body, over becoming pregnant. I'm proud of my decision to stop. Stopping fertility treatment was such a courageous thing to do, especially when the world we live in will have you believing otherwise.

Letting go also meant I could focus on my relationship with the man who patiently stood by my side for 10 years – we owed that to ourselves. It meant my husband and I, as a family of two, could focus on the dreams that only involved us. Many people say that part of healing is about finding meaning beyond parenthood, and I believe that too, but I use the term 'meaning' loosely. Maybe your 'meaning' is to be a stay-at-home rabbit mum, or maybe it's to write a book, or perhaps it's none of these things. Meaning is whatever you want it to be. Don't feel pressured to 'find your purpose' because you're childfree after infertility. You don't need to justify what your today and tomorrows look like.

Living a childfree life

I'm often asked what advice I would give others about navigating a childfree-after-infertility life. As a coach, I always say to my childfree clients, 'If we're always guided by other people's advice, what's the point in having our own opinions?'. Instead of giving advice to others, I usually explain what helped me to move forward. I support people to work through their own thought process and come to their own solutions.

I read an Instagram post that said: 'The quality of your healing can determine the way you live the rest of your life'. There are no truer words than those. This is why my path to healing was extensive and I approached it from many different angles:

Counselling – therapy was a game-changer for me. The fact that I was able to sit in my negative emotions and speak to someone who was completely objective about my feelings made a huge difference to my recovery and healing. I will always advocate for therapy as a strong component for dealing with loss, trauma and grief.

My faith – as a Muslim woman, I found a lot of comfort in praying and my belief in God. Hearing stories about highly revered, childfree women in my faith made me feel very empowered because I knew their lives had great purpose and meaning, way beyond motherhood. If their lives did, I knew that mine could too.

Coaching – this was so powerful. It helped me evaluate what was and wasn't important. It supported me in thinking about what I wanted to do for the rest of my life now that motherhood was no longer an option. It led me to leave my day job and quite literally create a life that I love. Becoming a coach and contributing to the online community feels like a dream come true. That was definitely the 'meaning' I wanted and needed in my life.

Finally, this might be a hard pill for some readers to swallow but, moving forward means taking responsibility for making the changes you want in your life. I was sick and tired of waking up feeling sad all day, every day, and I decided I wanted my life to look and feel different. The process definitely can't be rushed. Everyone has their own timeline when working through the grief and trauma they've experienced.

Reminder to wider society – we don't need to move forward on your timing, we will get through things when we are ready!

Debunking the childfree-after-infertility myth

Myth: a childfree-after-infertility life is an empty life. It really isn't. The messy part, as I explained above, is the transition. Once you've moved past the ache and accepted your reality, beautiful things await; however, you have to be willing to work at it. Finding happiness and acceptance doesn't mean that grief won't resurface. We all know the phrase, 'healing is not linear'. This is very true when embracing a childfree-after-infertility life. When grief does reappear, I greet her like an old friend – I acknowledge my thoughts and feelings and remind myself that they too, shall pass. Understandably, working through grief and trauma takes time but, at some point, even with the difficulties you've experienced, you will find joy again. Working through difficult emotions can feel like a huge weight has been lifted.

Eventually, my husband and I stopped feeling left behind really, we are just beginning. We realised that the world was our oyster, and with that in mind, we decided what our oyster would look like – refocusing on the important, yet simple things we had neglected during our trying-to-conceive years. We started spending more time with our friends and family, including our nephews, who we love deeply, but are thankful we can hand back at the end of the day (ha ha). We can now devote more quality time to our cat, Peaches, who we are so in love with – she loves not having to share our attention. We've been able to travel much more, and one of our favourite childfree perks is searching for childfree destinations, including hotels and restaurants. The freedom that our childfree life gives us is something my husband and I don't take for granted.

Support and acceptance about one's decision

I often receive DMs from people telling me that they don't know how much more they can keep trying but worry about 'giving up' because of what others will think. Will people think they didn't try hard enough, or didn't want it enough? It's never easy shrugging off the opinions of others – I'm at a place of contentment (thank goodness), but it hasn't always been this way. There's a huge stigma attached to being infertile, particularly in South Asian communities. Being half South Asian myself, I felt stigma from the wider South Asian community because I wasn't a mother. The infertility journey is hard enough without judgement from those around us. I want people reading this to know that it's okay if you feel like you don't belong, fit in or want to be around others who have children. These are legitimate feelings when being infertile and leaving the process childless. Some of these feelings may continue indefinitely.

A good support network

A good support network is essential for those quitting their infertility journey and about to embrace a childfree life. Accepting the reality of a situation can cause a lot of grief, trauma and upset, so it's completely normal to be sad about the life you wished for. Expect your healing journey to have bumps along the way – grief can often rear its ugly head at the most unexpected times. What's most needed from others during this period is acknowledgment and compassion while respecting your decision to stop. It's okay to create boundaries while you're trying to find your path towards a childfree-after-infertility life, in the same way you may have done when trying to conceive. Honouring your boundaries is crucial. You're letting others know that their lives are not more important than yours. The transition period may feel like you're re-entering society and starting over from scratch – these feelings are absolutely normal too.

Being around supportive people made a huge difference to my recovery. Find your community – there are plenty of people who want to support you, whether it's through the online community, workshops, or 1-2-1 coaching, we are out there.

We're a community – include us

I jumped at the chance to share my story when Lauren asked if I'd write a chapter for this book. The infertility community isn't always inclusive of stories like mine. I understand why, but it's important not to erase our voices from the infertility narrative. The reality is that many people who try to conceive naturally, or go through ART, won't end up with a baby. People who embrace a childfree-after-fertility life deserve space in this community too. After all, we are STILL infertile.

What can we all do to be more inclusive? Work with us and share our stories, especially if it's different to yours! Amplify our voices because we matter too. It can make all the difference when someone sees a post that includes their lived experience.

The journey I've been on has been extremely long and it feels amazing to finally be happy with the life I have now. It feels strange, reflecting on a time when coping looked like making it to the end of the day, day after day. What feels even more incredible is that my future plans include a whole heap of, 'whatever the heck I want'. *Smile*. Are there times when I am triggered? Of course! But these moments are few and far between and I believe this is normal for anyone who has been through experiences that are painful or meaningful to them.

The main reason why writing this chapter was hugely important to me was that my story might represent hope. A childfree-after-infertility life might not be one you planned, but it can definitely be full of happiness – I'm living proof of that.

Connect with me

I absolutely love coaching and I am deeply passionate about empowering those who want to live a richer, more fulfilling life. To find out more about the work I do, book a free discovery call or 1:1 coaching session – I'd love to connect with you.

Website: www.mindbodyrevivalcoach.com
Instagram: @mindbodyrevival_coach
Twitter: @mindbodyrevival
LinkedIn:
www.linkedin.com/company/mindbodyrevivalcoach

Chosen charity

Our charity is Tommy's: www.tommys.org

1 in 4 pregnancies end in loss or premature birth. Tommy's believe that every baby lost is one too many. They exist to support, care for and champion people, no matter where they may be on their pregnancy journey. It's a charity close to my heart because of the battles

I've had with my own pregnancy losses. Tommy's is there to help, and you can talk to a midwife for free, Monday-Friday, 9am-5pm. They can be contacted on 0800 0147 800 or emailed midwife@tommys.org. All their midwives are trained in bereavement support and will be able to talk to you about what you're going through.

Aideen and Andrew

Aideen and Andrew McCanny endured seven IVF transfers before falling pregnant with twins. After a complicated pregnancy, the twins were born via emergency c-section at 30 weeks. What followed was weeks spent in the NICU of two different hospitals. Following a severe infection, after seven weeks they lost their boy twin, Eoin, and just a few days later, they brought his sister Lucia home. Aideen is unexpectedly pregnant naturally with their rainbow baby and is due on her birthday in September 2021.

Aideen

I still remember that initial conversation well. We were in our favourite local coffee shop (which would become the scene for many more serious conversations over the years) and had been in our newlywed bubble for just three months. Before we got married, we decided we would have one more – what we called – 'blow-out year'. This would be a year for just us, to travel, enjoy time with friends and have as much fun as possible. However, curiosity perhaps, got the better of us. We decided we were ready to take that step into parenthood together.

The thing that I replay over and over in my head is how optimistic we were about it. We were young (26 and 27 at the time), fit and healthy with no known fertility 'issues' on either side of the family. We actually joked that we would be one of those couples who fell pregnant after just a month or two of trying. That's how sure we were about it.

The first year was pretty stress-free. The grip of infertility hadn't caught us just yet. There was plenty of socialising and trips, and Ovulation Predictor Kits hadn't yet become a part of our lives. But as we approached the end of the first year, believe it or not, despite being relaxed about it, nothing had happened. That niggling feeling started at the back of my mind that maybe something wasn't quite right. Friends who were married after us had started to announce their pregnancies and suddenly the question of 'Why not us?' began.

We discussed it and Andrew, being a doctor, was very level headed about it. He had no concerns and did well to ease my mind, something which he continues to do daily. I called my GP and booked an appointment. I was brought in for a full blood work up, which included a test to check if I was ovulating. A few days later, I received a phone call advising me that I needed to come back to see my doctor – cue panic. Most of the tests had come back normal, except my testosterone, which was slightly elevated. It later transpired this was, in fact, incorrect. My bloods had been taken at the wrong stage of my cycle and a repeat result on day 21 showed everything was normal. The next step was for Andrew to have a semen analysis carried out at our local hospital. Again, there were no issues there, plus I was ovulating and my AMH was normal, so why weren't we pregnant yet?!

A few months later, we received an appointment with a Consultant Gynaecologist at the fertility clinic in our local hospital. She could tell I was anxious about it but advised that it was still early days. We were young and so she suggested we go away and if in six months' time I wasn't yet pregnant, the next step would be to have further investigations, before being placed on the waiting list for IVF.

I tried to relax, I really did, but by this stage I was consumed by it all. I think once you begin the process of finding out if there could be a problem it takes over. I started counting down the time to appointments. That two-week wait every month was like a kick in the teeth. More friends and family members announced pregnancies, babies were being born and yet our lives seemed to be standing still. I felt so left out. We were ready for this to happen but we had no control over the situation.

I threw myself into work to keep busy. At the weekend we would venture to fancy hotels, I'd constantly treat myself to new clothes and dream about our next holiday, which was never too far away. Don't get me wrong, we had a great time and we have so many amazing memories but for me, it was always tinged with a little sadness. I knew we were lucky to be able to live our life this way, but I felt like I was just filling the void, waiting for when I would finally be pregnant.

Fast forward a few months and still nothing. I tried reflexology and sought the advice of a dietitian, changing my diet so it was considered more 'fertility friendly'. On the rare month when my period was late, I was always met with a single line or the words 'Not Pregnant' on pregnancy tests. Then the date for my hysteroscopy arrived. I was nervous and a bit angry, if I'm honest. I couldn't believe that I was having to put my body through surgery in order to find out why we couldn't get pregnant. It felt very much like the burden was on my shoulders. One single test showed there were no issues on Andrew's side, so the problem had to be with me. Still, if we got some answers, at least it would be a step in the right direction.

I woke up post-surgery dazed and confused. The consultant told me there were no issues. Everything looked normal. It was at this point we were given the dreaded 'unexplained infertility' diagnosis. There were no more tests that could be carried out. Our best chance at getting pregnant was IVF.

At this point, I think I had moved past anger. Infertility affects 1 in 8 couples and unfortunately, amongst our group of friends, the statistic landed on us.

But we had a solution: IVF. I knew little about it, apart from what I now know to be largely inaccurate portrayals in TV shows or films. I used the nine months that we were on the waiting list to educate myself on it. I bought books, immersed myself in medical websites online and actually became quite excited about it. I look back now and I can see how naïve I was. I'd adopted the same attitude I had when we started trying naturally. I was sure IVF would work first time. There were no obvious reasons why we weren't able to achieve a pregnancy ourselves so this was all that we needed to 'fix' whatever the problem was.

As a couple, we made the decision to be open with friends and family about what was happening. I, unashamedly, wear my heart on my sleeve. My emotions are out there for the world to see and I have the absolute worst poker face. We were over two and a half years into our marriage and were constantly getting the 'When are you going to start a family?' question. It hurt every time and my defence was to tell the person that we were on the waiting list for IVF. I thought that if I could make that person stop and think for a second before asking someone else this question, I would save them the same heartache we were enduring. That's one of the great lessons that infertility has taught me. Perhaps the old me, the one before any of this happened, would have unknowingly asked others this question. Now I know better.

For me – and I'm sure for many couples who are struggling to conceive – the hardest part of this process were the pregnancy announcements. I constantly reminded myself that the world wasn't going to stop having babies just because we weren't. This was our issue, not theirs. But it's hard when something you want so badly seems to come so easily to others. It wasn't that I wasn't happy for them – I really was. It was just that I was sad for me. There is such an injustice when it comes to infertility. It doesn't matter if you would make amazing parents or that you deserve this. Infertility isn't biased.

The biggest heartache for me was visiting friends after they had just brought their gorgeous bundles home. Shopping for baby clothes for someone else's baby, when you so want it to be for your own baby, comes with a whole wave of conflicting emotions.

I spent a lot of time worried about losing friends. Again, I think this was partly why we decided to be open about what was happening to us. I felt that if others knew what was happening, they would understand my strange behaviour and perhaps even excuse it. I'm so lucky that somehow, I managed to maintain those friendships. I think out of everything that has happened to us, I am most proud of this.

Finally, it seemed like all the waiting was over. We were at the top of the list for IVF. Our consultant explained that under the NHS in Northern Ireland, we were entitled to two free transfers. I was excited. Surely this was going to work!

We met with the nurse and received our drugs, schedule, education on how to administer daily injections, what pills to take and when, and when I'd need to attend for scans, bloods, etc. It was overwhelming but I knew we could handle it and I was very grateful that Andrew was a doctor. At this stage, there was also the novelty factor. This was something new to try and I had every faith in the process.

With our first cycle, everything was smooth – textbook in fact. I had 20 eggs collected and was on the cusp of having a freeze-all cycle but the consultant was happy for us to proceed with a fresh transfer. Those 20 eggs resulted in four grade B embryos. I was sure that at least one of them would be our baby.

The next 10 days were hell. Everyone who has been through IVF will tell you this is the worst part of the process. Daily injections are a breeze compared to the mental torture that ensues. Initially, I was optimistic. I felt pregnant. I let myself dream. And then I started to lightly spot, which eventually turned into bleeding. I somehow held off and waited until official test day but there it was: another blank screen with only a solo line staring back at me. I shrugged it off. It hadn't worked but that didn't mean it wouldn't. We had three more embryos waiting for us.

And so, I geared up for our first frozen embryo transfer. The NHS moves very slow so we had to wait a while before we could proceed. But finally, the date arrived when we could get started. We added in an endometrial scratch this time to try and increase our chances. An FET cycle is definitely physically a little easier but emotionally, it's just as hard. This time I didn't spot or bleed. Again, I held off until test day but the outcome was the same.

By this stage, I was beyond frustrated. We had good quality embryos, everything had gone smoothly, so why hadn't it worked? We met with our consultant for what is lovingly known in the IVF community as the WTF (What The F**k) meeting to discuss what was going on. Unsurprisingly, our consultant didn't have any answers for us. She actually said she expected it to have worked by now, which just made me feel worse. She told us about a trial that was happening in England, which checks levels of Natural Killer (NK) cells in the womb and suggested before we transfer any more embryos, to think about this. After looking into it, we decided to give it a go. I was confident that this was the reason my body was rejecting our precious embryos. If we could find the problem, we could fix it.

Two trips to England, two painful biopsies later and yet again, I was told there were no issues. We had used our two, free NHS cycles so if we wanted to proceed with IVF, we'd have to go private. We decided to stick with the same clinic, only this time we were paying. I was sure this would mean a quicker service and perhaps more attention to detail, but money means very little in this game. Despite handing over thousands of pounds, I still very much felt like a number.

Within another six months or so, we had another two failed FETs under our belt. I was at an all-time low. Upon reflection, I was probably depressed. I was finding it harder and harder to see a baby in our future. It was so frustrating that this had become so difficult for us. As a couple, we decided we needed a little break. We needed some time to get the money together to start a new cycle, and mentally, I needed to take a step back. I definitely didn't detach myself from the situation though. It was always on my mind. I was counting down the months until we could start again.

During this time, I threw myself into doing what I could to improve my mental wellbeing. I indulged in all the self-care possible and sought the services of a counsellor. For me, this was conflicting. It was good to have an hour a week dedicated to getting all my thoughts and feelings out there but more often than not, I would leave a session feeling worse than when I went in. The only time I felt in anyway optimistic was when I was going through the process of another IVF cycle, which sounds strange, but actively trying to fix the 'problem' made me feel like we were doing something about it.

I also decided to set up an Instagram account

dedicated to sharing our next IVF cycle. It was probably the best thing I did for my mental health. Feeling like I was part of a community of women, all going through the same thing, made me feel less lonely. At the time, we were the only couple in our friendship group going through IVF so I felt like no one really understood. But these ladies got it and they had a way of picking me up when I felt low. I followed loads of accounts of people who had gone through several cycles of IVF before getting pregnant. Finally, some of that optimism from the initial days had come back.

With the funds in hand, we decided it was time to change clinics; a fresh approach, and new surroundings, were exactly what we needed. In Northern Ireland, we have very little choice when it comes to clinics. At the time, there were in fact only two in the country. We had had no success with the first one so this very much felt like our last chance.

Our initial consultation went well. The consultant looked at our history and given the high number of eggs collected and huge drop off in fertilisation rates, he recommended ICSI. He also recommended a slightly lower dose of stims to avoid the dreaded OHSS, and if we were lucky to have two blastocysts, transferring them both together would be a good option for us. We were excited. A fresh perspective had led to some changes and I felt good about it.

The cycle went well with no major issues. I felt a bit more at ease this time as I knew what to expect. I was also thrilled that I'd be sedated for egg collection – a luxury which, unfortunately, the NHS were unable to offer me. I woke up groggy, to the consultant telling me they had retrieved 18 eggs.

The next day, any happiness I felt soon dissipated following a phone call with the embryologist. Out of 18 eggs, 10 were mature and six had fertilised. This sounded good to me but the concern in the embryologist's voice told me there was more to this call. I was told that out of these six eggs, four of them were dark and 'grainy' in the centre. This led to a discussion about how my eggs are unique because they don't all possess this structure, but it was likely that poor egg quality was a factor. It felt like a slap in the face. All these years I had wanted to know what the issue was and now that I knew it was down to my crappy eggs and there was nothing I could do about it, I was devastated.

Over the next few days, I tried not to focus on these findings and instead keep at the forefront of my mind that we were still creating day 5 embryos, so surely that was a good sign?! On the morning of transfer, we received a phone call to say we had one grade A and one grade B embryo. Both the embryologist and consultant recommended just transferring one this time and given that we had never had an A grade embryo before, we were happy with this advice.

Another dreaded two-week wait followed. I didn't make it to test day this time without bleeding. I knew it was over a few days before our official test day. I was gutted. The nurse at the clinic was devastated when I went in for my Beta test and told her I had tested negative. It genuinely seemed like everyone around us wanted this for us. We waited a couple of months and transferred our one remaining embryo. The outcome was the same.

We now had six failed transfers behind us. I was really struggling to see how this would ever work for us. Still, I wasn't ready to give up. We decided to go with one more cycle. In my mind, I had already decided what we would do next. When I learned that poor egg quality was most likely the issue, I couldn't think about anything else. I started following accounts of other women who'd had success using donor eggs. Andrew would get frustrated by my negative attitude but he let me do what I needed to do in order to get through this. I had found a clinic abroad which offered donor egg cycles and was adamant that if our next batch of embryos didn't work, this was our next step.

We again met with the consultant to discuss our options. As my AMH was on the higher side and I therefore tended to have a large number of eggs collected, it was recommended that I resume a lower dose of stims, over a longer period of time. The hope here was that they would retrieve less eggs, but the quality would be better.

By this stage, I felt like a pro. I had lost count of how many pills I'd popped and injections I had given myself. Scans and blood tests had become a way of life and I muddled through it. Some of that optimism was still there and I think this is what carried me through. However, things didn't really go to plan this time. Despite the change in protocol, I had loads of follicles. I was also told that my oestradiol reading was through the roof. I was told to come into the clinic as soon as possible to collect medication to try to prevent OHSS and I would need to trigger that night. This also meant that this would be a freeze-all cycle. I would need to let my ovaries calm down for a couple of months and transfer a frozen embryo instead.

I was terrified that this earlier-than-planned collection would mean a high number of immature eggs, so I was pleasantly surprised to hear that we had 16, 10 of which were mature and we ended up with three grade A and three grade B's in the freezer.

This had, by far, been my most stressful stims cycle

to date, so much so that I felt I needed a break. I was physically and mentally exhausted and so, we decided to leave those lovely little embryos in the freezer and head off on holiday before Christmas, then start the FET process all over again when we returned.

This time, we decided to transfer two embryos. I was deflated at this point and this was the only way I could see us increasing what little chance we had. We had six frozen embryos and the thought of transferring them all individually made me feel exhausted. There was no way I could face six more transfers. On the morning of transfer, the embryologist called with more bad news. It looked like one of the embryos hadn't thawed well. She said we should prepare ourselves for a single transfer. I was frustrated but I had learned to accept that nothing is predictable in this game. However, when we arrived at the clinic, we were told that it had bounced back and was good to be transferred, along with our other grade A.

Our seventh two-week wait ensued. My strategy was always to stay busy. I cooked, cleaned and distracted myself as much as possible. Our official test day was at 12dp5dt, which was a Monday. I was so sure we were facing another negative result that I decided to test on the Friday night – the reasoning being that we would have the weekend to come to terms with it.

I can't quite put into words how I felt when that plus sign appeared. In five years and seven rounds of IVF, it was the first positive pregnancy test that I held in my hands. We couldn't believe it. I spent the next few days in denial, sure that it wasn't true, but thankfully, on the Monday a strong Beta result confirmed that we were definitely, 100 per cent pregnant.

Anyone who has experienced pregnancy after infertility will undoubtedly tell you that the first trimester is rough. I think when you become accustomed to things going wrong for so long you expect the worst.

At seven weeks, I had a light bleed. Andrew was on-call so I was home alone. I called the on-call consultant at our clinic who told me that if it became heavy, I would need to go to the hospital. If it settled, he would see me in the morning for a scan. Spending the night on my own was awful. I hardly slept and was constantly running to the toilet to check if the bleeding had stopped. There hadn't been any more and I tried to tell myself that bleeding in early pregnancy was common but there was a voice in my head telling me that this was too good to be true. Good things just don't seem to happen to us.

Andrew arrived home from work early the next morning and we headed to the clinic. The consultant was in the middle of an egg retrieval and I paced the waiting room for an hour, trying not to be sick. I have never been so scared in my life. When it was finally time to be scanned, I was warned that it was still early days and we might not be able to see anything at this stage, but there it was – a tiny little baby with a beating heart. I asked if there was just one, to which the consultant replied that he thought he had seen a second sac. He moved the probe to the right and there it was: our second little baby, with its heart beating away. I burst into tears. Was this really happening?! After all this time, was I actually pregnant with not one, but two babies? I felt like finally, our luck had changed and we were being rewarded for everything we had been through.

Seeing those heartbeats early made me relax a little but I think it's safe to say I was on edge for the entire pregnancy. At my 12-week booking appointment, the consultant highlighted the risks of a twin pregnancy. She told me that 15% of twins are born before 32 weeks, a statistic I was shocked to hear. Still, I tried not to think too much of it. I had waited an eternity to be pregnant and I was going to enjoy this as much as I could. I ate well, walked daily, drank water by the bucketload, practiced yoga and enjoyed plenty of down time. I was feeling good and enjoying seeing my bump get bigger by the day. But at the back of my mind, something was telling me that I wouldn't make it to 37 weeks, so much so that I nested early. I made sure the nursery was complete, packed my hospital bag early, we had purchased everything we needed and I read every book on twins that I could find.

At around 28 weeks, things started to go wrong. I was constantly in pain; I couldn't sit or lie in the same position for longer than 20 minutes and I was surviving on just a few hours' sleep at night. Still, I told myself that this was all fine; that pregnancy was hard and these were all complaints I was happy to have.

A week or so later, I suddenly developed itching on my hands and feet. A quick Google search offered cholestasis as a diagnosis and so I called the hospital. The condition affects around 1 in 140 pregnant women and is caused when bile acids do not flow properly from the liver and build up in the body instead. I was told to come in for monitoring of the babies and some blood tests, which confirmed that I had, in fact, developed the condition. I was prescribed medication to try and reduce bile acid levels and was told to return to the hospital weekly for monitoring. I left with a warning to keep a close eye on babies' movements and call straight away if I had any concerns.

At my next monitoring appointment, another blood test showed that my bile acid levels had reduced but the concern now was about my kidney function. I was told to come in on Sunday for more bloods. That morning, as I was getting ready to go to my appointment, I felt a huge gush as my waters broke. In that moment, adrenaline took over. I called my husband, who was on-call and he told me to ring the hospital. I was told to come straight in. I was concerned about driving so my mother-in-law drove me there, which turned out to be a good idea as I started having contractions on the way.

By the time I was being assessed, I knew I was in labour. I was brought up to the delivery suite to try and stop things but at this stage, I was already over 5cm dilated. To make things worse, I was told that the NICU didn't have two cots available and that I might be transferred to another hospital. However, when the consultant went to examine me again, twin A was really low down and basically on the way out so the ambulance was cancelled. An hour later, I was 10cm dilated and felt ready to start pushing but twin A's cord had prolapsed.

Before I knew it, I was being rushed down a corridor into a theatre. There were about 10 people in the room. I kept asking where Andrew was but before I could even process what was happening, I was given general anaesthetic.

The consultant said it was one of the quickest sections she had ever performed, with both babies being born in the exact same minute. Because twin A was so low down, she had to remove twin B first in order to make room to scoop twin A out of my pelvis. I woke up to Andrew telling me that we had a son and a daughter, and I was wheeled up to NICU to meet them. We named them Eoin and Lucia.

I wish I could say that this was the end of our story but really, our heartache had only just started. What followed was weeks spent in the NICU of two hospitals. Initially, things were going well. Both babies were making progress and we were counting down the days until we got to bring them home. However, Eoin contracted NEC – a severe infection in the bowel, which sadly is common in premature babies. He seemingly started to get better, before we were told he needed emergency surgery. He was transferred to a different hospital, which meant we were dividing our time between both babies, which is the worst thing you could ask any parent to do. A week after Eoin's initial surgery, he was back in theatre again but this time, we were met with the words: 'There is nothing we can do'. In that second, I couldn't breathe. I couldn't understand how our little boy, so full of life and fight, could be taken from us.

Just a couple of days later, Eoin took his last breath. And a few days after that, we brought his sister Lucia home.

Losing a twin is devastating. It's a strange kind of grief and unlike anything I've ever experienced before. 'How are you?' is a question I'm asked daily and there's no straightforward way to answer it. The truth is, I don't really know how I am. It's a conflicting thing to feel heartbroken and happy all at once; my heart aches for Eoin, yet I'm overjoyed every time I look at Lucia.

The loss of a twin is a whole new type of grief. It's hard to describe. I question everything I do. I get dressed and put makeup on as usual every day, which is something I questioned when someone commented that I 'look well considering'. It made me wonder if I'm not grieving in the typical way you would expect, but then again, these aren't normal circumstances.

I've learned never to judge someone's grief. We're living our lives as normal as possible because we have to for Lucia. To the outsider, it looks like we have it pretty good. Friends and family came to visit us and we've laughed and enjoyed doing all the typical things you do when you bring a new baby home. We've loved every second of having Lucia home but that doesn't mean that inside we aren't aching. I spend much of the day thinking about Eoin and how different things would be if he was still here, how he and his sister would interact and who he would look like. I worry so much about how we'll tell Lucia about all of this when she's older. I fear that she will always feel like part of her is missing. I want nothing but a happy life for her because she deserves this after the start that she had.

During my pregnancy, I planned a future for them. Everything was done in twos. Our nursery was decorated for these two babies, we bought a double pram, read all the books on what to do when you're having two, and even bought a bigger car. The hardest thing was modifying those plans to suit just one.

Lucia is now seven months old (four months corrected) and she is a happy, content little baby. She brings so much happiness to our lives during a time when we need it the most. When she's older, she will know all about her little brother and what a fighter he was. I have no doubt that some of his strength and determination will live on in her. Earlier, I mentioned that on our transfer day, one of those embryos bounced back and was suitable for transfer. In seeing how strong he was, I have no doubt that that embryo was Eoin.

I think that if this whole journey has taught me anything, it's to expect the unexpected. As I sit here writing this, I am currently 12 weeks pregnant with our rainbow baby, due on my birthday in September 2021.

We actually discussed doing IVF again in the future, so to be pregnant now and know that Lucia will have a sibling close to her age is absolutely wonderful. We are so happy that our family is growing. To be pregnant naturally after everything we have been through was totally unexpected and we are very grateful for the little bit of good fortune that has come our way.

This pregnancy won't be without its challenges but I'm learning to take it one day at a time. In amongst the disbelief and happiness, there have been lots of questions, fear and 'what ifs'. I've learnt that pregnancy after baby loss definitely comes with a new wave of emotions.

I often get asked how I proceeded with so many IVF cycles and what I did to stay positive. I don't have any magic solution that is going to get you through this any easier, but all I can offer is hope. If you'd told me 10 years ago all that we would go through, I definitely wouldn't have believed you. While our story is one of loss, more than anything, I want it to be one of optimism. Hope was all we had and going forward with this pregnancy, hope is all we have now. I hope that things will be different this time because I need this baby to be born healthy and well, not just for him or her but for us too.

Connect with me on Instagram: @ivfmumblings

Chosen charity

Our charity is Tiny Life:
www.tinylife.org.uk

They're a premature baby charity in Northern Ireland, who help families with premature or unwell newborns. They provide support services both in the Neonatal Unit and in the community.

Claire

After a diagnosis of PCOS (polycystic ovary syndrome) at an early age, Claire was told she couldn't have children. In her thirties, she decided to embark upon a SMBC (single mother by choice) journey to have a baby. She talks about her experience with PCOS, making the decision to pursue treatment, choosing a donor and failed cycles.

Claire

My name is Claire, I'm 38 and I'm currently embarking on my journey to become a single mother by choice (SMBC). I always knew I wanted to be a mother, either on my own or with a partner. My journey has been relatively short so far, but not without its challenges.

For me, my journey began when I was 10. That is the age I got my first period. When I turned 12, my problems began. My cycle became extremely frequent. I was getting a period every 22 days and it would last at least 12 days, meaning I was bleeding almost constantly. At 12, the pain started. I began having severe pain in my lower abdomen and groin, particularly on my right side. My GP put me on a 'light' pill to control the cycle and the pain. For two years, I had numerous investigations performed to establish what this pain was. They removed my appendix – which, as it turned out, was normal. I had three exploratory laparoscopies done, all with no real answer as to the cause of this pain and frequent periods. I didn't take painkillers because they didn't help and firmly believed then, as I do now, that analgesia should only be used if and when they are helping.

The only answers I was offered were the following diagnoses by a gynaecologist. I was told I had salpingitis, which is inflammation of the fallopian tubes caused by infection and that this would cause scarring of the tubes – which would mean I wouldn't be able to have children. I was told this by a male gynaecologist, who stood at the end of my hospital bed and showed no compassion whatsoever while he told me this. As a nurse myself, I can categorically say this should never have happened like this. The correct investigations had not been performed to diagnose this.

I was then told it was ovulation pain and if the pill didn't help, I'd have to get used to it. The final diagnosis came when I was 13. I was told by the same gynaecologist that I had 'multiple cysts on my ovaries instead of eggs'. He again reiterated this would mean that as I wouldn't be able to release an egg, I wouldn't be able to have children of my own. I later learned that this was PCOS (polycystic ovary syndrome). It was 1995 so I'm not sure that it had a name at the time or if he just didn't bother to tell me what it was. He put me on Dianette® and I remained on this for the next 24 years, until I started my IVF cycle. This helped with the pain and it more or less disappeared. The news that I may never have children devastated me at the time but I was so young, and my mother is such a caring, typically Irish mammy, that she assured me that it was 'a might, not a definite'. Although it was still there, I put it to the back of my mind as much as I could.

When I was 16, I made the distressing discovery that the hair on my head was falling out, to the point that my scalp was becoming visible, and I was growing hair on my breasts. I eventually confided in my mother. We spoke at length about it and how distressed I had become due to this. She admitted that she had noticed it but didn't want to upset me by bringing it up until I was ready to discuss it. We agreed that I would attend our GP and discuss it with her.

I attended the GP on my own and told her what was going on. At the start, she was very professional. She examined my scalp and asked the appropriate questions to establish if it was alopecia. She then blew up my whole world. She told me I had polycystic ovary syndrome. She explained that this meant I produced cysts where my eggs should be. She told me in no uncertain terms that I was infertile and would never be able to have children. I don't know if it was because I was a bit older or because this was the third time in three years I'd heard it, but I was inconsolable. She advised me to stay on my pill and lose weight (of note, my weight was not normal at the time but I wasn't obese by any stretch of the imagination).

The walk home from the GP was the longest walk of my life. I was happy to have a name for what was wrong with me, but I had no answer for what to do about the hair loss on my head or the hair growth on my breasts. I hadn't been offered any hope for my fertility. I certainly wasn't given any information on the condition to help me understand it or what to expect going forward. By the time I got home, I was so upset I could barely speak. My mother spoke to the GP, who told her that if I wanted, she'd refer me to a gynaecologist but that they'd tell me the same as she had. I attended a different gynaecologist and he did tell me the same, except that he told me to come back to him when I wanted to start trying for a family.

The hair on my head remains extremely thin, to the point that I now use a scalp concealer, hair fibres and clip-in hair extensions to make me look like I have more hair than I do. This is a daily chore but it has improved my life completely – I could never go back to having my scalp so exposed. This, however, presents its own problems. For example, when I lie down on the examination couch in the clinic for a scan, I am acutely aware that my 'hair' is probably coming off and will be all over the protective sheet on the couch. To save embarrassment, I then have to scramble when I'm getting dressed to remove this. Another time that I'm extremely aware of the fake hair is when I hug somebody, because the fibres can be left on the other person's face. PCOS is more than just being overweight and having hair on your face, as many people think.

When I was about 28, another GP in my practice decided that because I suffer with migraines, it was no longer suitable for me to stay on Dianette®, as this can cause migraine. She put me on Metformin and referred me to a gynaecologist who had an interest in PCOS. This appointment was very different to my previous gynaecologist appointments. She properly explained PCOS to me, with the knowledge that I'm a nurse and can understand the lingo, as well as explaining why Metformin works. She assured me that I would be able to have children but that I'd need 'a lot of help from IVF'. Even though this wasn't the news I was hoping for, it at least gave me a small glimmer of hope!

About a year later, I was on both Dianette® and Metformin and I started bleeding again between withdrawal periods. I attended my gynaecologist once more and she performed a Hysterosalpingograph (HSG) and D&C. She assured me that my tubes were clear and that it was highly unlikely that I'd ever had salpingitis. She felt that the bleeding between periods was from my lining not fully shedding and that the D&C would help, and after a couple of months, it did.

I have the worst taste in men. I always knew this and I think this contributed to my decision to become a SMBC. When I was 19, I decided that I was going to be a mother, regardless of my circumstances or the predictions of gynaecologists during my teen years. If I'm being completely honest, even from a young age I thought I'd be a single mother! I don't know why, but I did. When I got to about 23, I started looking into the options I would have to become a single mother. I always knew that IVF would be an option and possibly my only chance of carrying a baby. I looked into adoption, but in Ireland there are no domestic adoptions really. They are primarily grandparent adoptions or adoptions from foster care. I then researched overseas adoption and became quite well versed on the process, but it is extremely expensive and was out of my reach at that stage. I began saving for my journey, as well as for a home, as I was renting with friends at the time.

At 27, I bought a home on my own. After a couple of years, I again began to look into overseas adoption. Things had changed and a lot of countries had closed to overseas adoption, and I was advised that those that were open would favour couples, as opposed to single women. I resigned myself that this would probably not be my path to motherhood. The drive to become a mother never left me though.

In my early thirties, I looked into fostering. I knew that I could provide a loving home for a child and hoped that this would happen. I spoke to my cousin, who is a social worker, and she advised me that it is an extremely difficult road, and that the emotional toll it takes when the child leaves is huge. With all this knowledge, I made initial enquiries to become a foster parent. I was rejected. The reply was simple and avoided saying that it was because I was single. Instead, they told me that they require one of the foster parents to be at home at all times. By this stage, I was a Clinical Nurse Manager (ward sister) and worked full time (which I still do), however as a CNM, I no longer worked nights so I thought that I might be eligible. I had explained that my mother would be the only other care provider, and that I worked until 6pm four days a week, therefore a school-age child would only be with my mother for three hours. I was devastated.

Although the urge, want and need to become a mother never left me, I put active attempts to pursue it on the backburner slightly... until I turned 36 and I could no longer quieten the need to have a child. I had spoken openly to family and friends about my want to become a mother and that IVF was most likely to be my route to realising this. My parents weren't unsupportive at all, but they felt that I still had time to meet someone and do things the 'traditional' way. As I'd be on my own, I'd need my parents' support in this, especially when it came to childcare. I needed them to be on board and be ready. Also, I didn't have the money to pursue IVF at that time.

When I turned 37, I decided I wasn't waiting any longer and told my family that this was the year I was finally going to start IVF. It took some time for them to come to terms with it but they were always supportive. In December 2019, I was talking to my father about something random and I told him my name for a baby boy; he said to me, 'If your mam and I had had a boy, that was our name as well'. I don't know why but that conversation felt like a sign to go ahead! I'd been debating attending a fertility fair information day that my now-clinic were holding in January 2020. I made the decision there and then to attend and asked my mother to come with me and to be my support during the journey. She was so supportive and agreed without hesitation. We spoke about it afterwards and when I asked what changed, she simply said, 'You seem ready now and none of us are getting any younger, I want to be a grandmother'. I'm the eldest of four girls so there's still plenty of time for them, but I appreciated the honesty, as always. I also discussed it with the rest of my family that day and they were, and indeed still are, my biggest supporters.

On 26th January 2020, I attended the fertility information day and gained a huge amount of knowledge. This day, along with speaking to a friend that had worked for the clinic in a different part of the country, solidified my decision to proceed with my now-clinic. I found this information day extremely helpful. They discussed the treatment options for single women, heterosexual couples and same-sex couples. They also had a talk from their nutritionist, which I found very helpful and I used this service when I joined the clinic. I completed an appointment request form on the day. When I got home from this very informative day, I started a journal to my baby. In it, I tell them everything that is happening along the journey. I love to read back on it and I'm so happy I've done it.

I had more decisions than just which clinic to pick, of course. I had to try and come up with the money for the treatment. In Ireland, IVF is roughly €5000 a cycle and given that I am on my own, I'd need to buy sperm as well. I had some savings but decided to borrow €15,000 to give me three full cycles, if needed (I was afraid I wouldn't get any embryos due to my PCOS).

The process for accessing fertility treatment in Ireland is pretty simple; you can either self-refer or be referred by your GP. In general, couples struggling to conceive would have a GP referral that would outline previous investigations etc. I self-referred, as I felt I knew my history better than my GP. In Ireland, there is no financial support for fertility treatments and we are not given any free cycles or investigations. If you have health insurance, they may cover the cost of some treatment. For example, my insurer will grant €1000 once in a life time for fertility treatment – as previously mentioned, an IVF cycle will cost approximately

€5000.

You can claim back tax on all medical expenses, including fertility treatment, but if granted, this is only 20% of the final amount. One benefit that does help greatly is that you can access a drug payment scheme (DPS). This is a scheme whereby you pay €114 a month, no matter the cost of the meds. All are eligible, you just have to apply. There are very few fertility clinics in Ireland, I think there are six, and two satellite clinics that only do bloods and scans for their parent clinics. This poses huge logistical problems at times – I myself had to leave my house at 6am for an 8am scan appointment numerous times. Don't get me wrong, I'd travel to the ends of the earth and back if I had to, but it doesn't make the process very user friendly.

In February 2020, I received a call from one of the patient coordinators, asking me to complete an appointment request form – which asks for more details than the form I'd completed at the fertility day. I did this and my appointment was booked in March 2020. When the appointment was made, I told my closest friends, who have been extremely supportive.

On the day of my appointment, my youngest sister drove myself, my mother and my second youngest sister to the appointment. My mother attended the appointment with me – my family's support has been amazing. I was a little emotional sitting in the waiting room, chatting to my mother, as I couldn't quite believe that I was actually doing it. I had spoken about it for so long, I was so happy to finally be doing something so proactive.

I was instantly comfortable with my consultant. I told her my story and she asked me if I had thought about which treatment option I'd prefer. I told her I'd like to go straight to IVF, given my age (37) and my

333

PCOS. She agreed and told me she was hopeful I wouldn't have too much difficulty. She talked me through the process in full detail, diagrams included. She advised me that I would require bloods and an SIS procedure (saline infusion sonohysterography – to check my uterus and endometrial cavity).

I expressed my concern regarding my weight, as I am 4ft 10 and, at the time, was 13st 7lb, so I asked if I could meet with the nutritionist. A referral was put on the system for the nutritionist to contact me. The consultant told me that she predicted I'd be at egg retrieval by May! I had the bloods done that day and I met with one of the clinic nurses. The nurse talked me through the process of using donor sperm, time lines and the legal requirement for implications counselling when using a donor. I then met with a patient coordinator, who took me through the pricelist and any extra expenses I could expect, she also advised me about the DPS. From the bloods taken that day, I was told my AMH was 21.6, which was fine.

In March 2020, I set up my SMBC Instagram page. I had been looking this up on my regular page for a number of months and finally got brave enough to do it. I spoke to my sisters about it and we agreed that they wouldn't follow me on that page just yet. I wanted to shout from the rooftops about what I was doing, but at the same time, a friend that had been through the IVF process with her husband told me that when other people know about your journey, you have to manage their expectations too. I have found this SMBC/IVF community an absolute fount of knowledge and support. I have connected with people all over the world that I can ask anything to and we check in with each other regularly. The knowledge I have gained has been invaluable. Like all social media, some people appear to be more concerned with the number of followers rather than their journey – for example, one woman I follow stated she was disappointed that announcing her BFP overshadowed getting to a certain amount of followers! Similarly some people, for whatever reason, are vicious towards others – thankfully, I haven't experienced this. Instead of taking either of these types of people to heart, my advice would be: if you are getting abuse or encountering unkind people, put your profile on private. If people's priorities seem so different to yours that it bothers you, remember that it says more about them than you, and we can always 'unfollow'.

And then the global pandemic hit.

On 16th March 2020, my clinic closed due to the COVID-19 pandemic, as recommended by ESHRE. I was absolutely devastated. After waiting so long to finally do this, I was on hold indefinitely. My struggle and heartbreak did not compare to those that were at transfer stage though, who didn't get to proceed. My heart broke for these people and my Instagram account was flooded with people dealing with this awful setback.

In April, I had my very in-depth tele-appointment with the clinic nutritionist. She made a lot of recommendations which I took on board. I had a lot of changes to make to my diet and to try and control my IBS (irritable bowel syndrome). As a nurse, I already knew the importance of gut health for overall health, however I was surprised by the importance for fertility. It was a hard road but I have made a lot of changes, even though my weight continues to be an issue, it has improved. It's a fantastic service and I'd recommend anybody who's offered the service within their clinic to utilise it – not just for weight loss but for absorption and overall health and nutrition.

As we were in lockdown at the time, the counsellor the clinic uses was closed and was not willing to do a tele-appointment. I eventually had my counselling appointment in May 2020 – it went well and she signed me off.

I used the time the clinic was closed to choose my sperm donor. My clinic uses Cryos International sperm bank. When I started searching, I was overwhelmed to say the least! I started looking at the website and saw you could filter by preferences. I started inputting the features in men I would naturally be physically attracted to, I don't know why but it just felt right for me to do it! I wasn't very specific, just hair and eye colour, both of which are the same as my own. You also have to pick your country of treatment and here in Ireland, we can only use non-anonymous donors so that filtered it even more. It still left me with about 200 potential donors. When I was going through the profiles, I printed ones that appealed to me. I then went through them again and looked at family history, which I think is important.

The clinic includes a letter from the donor on the profile, and you can also hear them reading it. The donors that stuck out for me were the ones who addressed that letter to the baby that would hopefully result from their donation. This became a real deciding factor for me! Donors that had children themselves also stood out. How they came across when answering the questions showed their personality to me, so I shortlisted again. There's no real science to it, I just did it in a way that felt right to me.

Then I asked my mother and sisters to look at the shortlisted donors, which helped hugely! Mam picked donors who looked like me as a baby, and based on the letter and personality. One of my sisters was willing to give her opinion, and she based her pick on the overall profile, the letter and baby pictures' likeness to our family. My other two sisters looked at them but felt it was a decision for me to make and my dad wasn't comfortable with knowing about the donor side of things (he is hugely supportive of me doing this though!) which I respected. When I took my mam and my sister's opinions into account, I was left with six profiles – the clinic required a selection of five donors, so it worked out great! The donor I had put as number three was available and he is my donor.

The clinic finally reopened in May 2020. They were very busy, as you can expect. I contacted them to schedule my SIS procedure and I was booked in for June. This is a procedure in which the doctor uses vaginal ultrasound and a saline solution to measure the direction and length of the entrance to the womb. This helps decide which type of catheter is needed and the depth at which the embryo should be inserted for transfer. Just as importantly, it assesses the uterus and fallopian tubes for any abnormalities, such as polyps, fibroids or tube blockage. My doctor advised me prior to the procedure that if there was an issue with the tubes, they generally recommend removal or ligation. I was shocked but as she said to me, I was doing IVF so it didn't mean infertility. The SIS was painless; I had some cramping but nothing too bad. When the fluid was inserted into my left tube I was quite uncomfortable but it's all worth it.

The good news was that everything looked fine. My left ovary looked very good. My right ovary was typically PCOS-looking, as in it had the pearl necklace appearance. My tubes were clear and no abnormalities were found in my uterus. This appointment was so different to the previous ones, as all appointments were limited to the person being treated only, and that remains the case at present.

In June 2020, I had my planning appointment and I couldn't wait to start treatment. The doctor informed me I'd be following a short, antagonist cycle, which tends to work best for PCOS. They also told me it would be six weeks before my chosen donor sperm would arrive at the clinic. I paid for the donor sperm the following day – €1300, including shipping, for one vial. It arrived at the end of July, so I could start my cycle on 13th August. I was elated.

I received my full outline and prescription by email and immediately dropped it to my local pharmacy. All my medications were ready two days before treatment started. I was shocked by the sheer volume of them and so excited to start. All my family came to my home to see the meds (again, I can't express how supportive my family and friends have been).

It felt like the 13th August would never come, but it did, and I had my first ever baseline scan. This is also one of my sisters' birthdays so I'll never forget it. All looked good and I was cleared to start my stims on the 15th August – which is the date of another of my sisters' birthdays, so after we got back from dinner that evening, I went to my parents' house and took my first batch of stims injections.

All my scans and bloods looked good over the next couple of weeks and my egg retrieval was booked for the 27th August. I was nervous, as I always had a fear that I wouldn't get any eggs due to my PCOS. The stimulation process was not easy. For me, the injections were the easiest part. I got so bloated and tired, and I had the sensation that I could feel my ovaries. I couldn't sit with my legs crossed or bend forward as it was extremely uncomfortable. My ovaries responded well though and I had 22 follicles that were all good sizes.

I took my dual trigger shots 36 hours before the retrieval. I had two shots to take at the same time, so I did one and my youngest sister did the other. She's a nurse as well and lives with me while she saves for the deposit for a house. During all my cycles, she's helped me so much – from emotional support to physically giving me most of the injections.

I was nervously excited to have my egg retrieval. I had to fast for four hours before the procedure but given that my appointment was for 8am, I fasted from midnight. I arrived at the clinic about 20 minutes before the appointment. With the new Covid restrictions, I had to wait in the car until I was contacted by the clinic. It was upsetting having to go in alone as I'd been told at the start of the journey that my mother could be with me. Everything has changed but hopefully not forever. When I entered the clinic, I had my IV line inserted and changed into my gown and socks (warm feet help to have a warm uterus). I then signed my consent with my doctor, and my nurse talked me through the discharge instructions. Next, I walked into theatre and positioned myself on the trolley with my legs in the now-familiar stirrups. After a bit more discussion as to what would happen while I was sedated, I drifted off to a blissful sleep.

When I awoke, I was pain free and well rested. I had a decaf coffee, as I'd switched in May to decaf and gave up alcohol (not that I drank much). After coming around a bit more, the doctor told me the great news – they had retrieved 22 eggs! I couldn't believe it. That was the good news, the bad news was that the clinic's policy is to freeze all if more than twenty eggs are retrieved, as this can be indicative of OHSS. I was absolutely devastated. This meant I'd have to wait at least another month, if not two, before I had my transfer. Everyone in the clinic were very kind and reassuring as always but my heart broke with the news. I was discharged and told that I'd receive a call from the embryology lab the following morning to let me know how many had fertilised. I must be very sensitive to the sedation as I slept for 24 hours after the procedure, only waking to eat or drink. I had no pain that day.

Bright and early the following morning, I answered the much-awaited call from the embryologist, who told me that 19 eggs had fertilised! I was shocked but absolutely delighted. Cue the longest weekend wait ever, as the next update wouldn't be until the Wednesday to let me know how many embryos were suitable for freezing. Over the next few days, I developed a lot of abdominal discomfort. I emailed the clinic and was scheduled for a scan on the Tuesday. My ovaries were still very large and were sitting on top on my uterus, causing the pain. I was happily reassured that all was well and was told that when my period started, the pain would go and indeed, on the Friday, this happened. The call on Wednesday from the embryologist went amazingly well. They had frozen eight day-5 blastocysts. As I've said before and during the journey to this stage, I was terrified that my egg quality or lack of eggs would mean that I wouldn't get embryos. This call healed my heart a little.

That same day, I had an unexpected call from my doctor to plan my frozen embryo transfer (FET). She also told me my embryos were all very good grades – a mix of AA, AB and BB. I had my next scheduling appointment in September and my FET was planned for my October cycle. As this was an FET, there were no injections this time, just oral medication to start with. After nearly two weeks of these, I had my ultrasound scan and was devastated to learn that my uterine lining was only 3.5mm. In order for an embryo transfer to go ahead, the lining should be 7mm at the very least. I was started on estrogen patches and my oral estrogen dose was increased.

I asked and was told that my lining at egg retrieval was only 4.5mm, which I assume means that even if they hadn't cancelled due to the large amount of eggs, it would have been cancelled due to the lining. I had a scan scheduled as part of my plan for the 12th October and I was advised to try not to worry. This was said with the best intentions and kindness but there was also a lot going on at the time – my neighbour's home heating oil leaked into my garden and the damage meant I had to move out of my house for a year. So worry and stress were already there.

At the next scan, my lining was only 4.5mm. My cycle was cancelled. I found this very hard to cope with. I became hugely disillusioned after this. I felt that I would never achieve my dream.

My next doctor's appointment was at the end of October. She was very positive and had a full plan, which included adding a blood thinning injection every day, medication to help blood flow and supplements proven to help with thin uterine lining. I also read online that lying on your left side and using a hot water bottle on the lower abdomen can help with blood supply to the uterus. I am willing to try everything and will do all this again before my next transfer (I won't use the hot water bottles afterwards though, as the embryos don't like heat). This all worked and I finally reached the magic number of 7mm for my FET, which happened on the 16th December 2020. Again, I was on my own, which I found so hard as I'd had my heart set on my mother being with me during all my appointments, but especially this day. The 16th December is my maternal grandmother's anniversary so we had a lot of hope that it was a sign. One of my sisters gave me an early Christmas present the day before the transfer of a good luck elephant figurine – to explain, I have always been obsessed with elephants, I feel they are my spirit animal.

On the day of transfer, I had to pass urine an hour before the appointment time then drink 750ml-1L of fluid – this is so the bladder is full. For the transfer, the ultrasound is conducted abdominally so the bladder must be full in order to visualise the uterus this way. When I arrived, my doctor went through the procedure and I signed my consent, changed into my gown and socks and entered theatre. In theatre, I got a bit emotional – as I sat onto the trolley my beautiful, perfect embryo popped up on the screen. Just seeing it up there on the screen gave me such hope and I felt a surge of love. I know this may seem like a strange thing to say, but I've wanted this for so long and was so invested in it. Without even trying, to this day I can still see that perfect embryo on the screen when I close my eyes.

When I sat on the trolley, the embryologist introduced herself and explained her role. My doctor again took me through what would happen during the transfer. Before the transfer begins, they check that you are who you're supposed to be and compare that with the details on the embryo. After these checks, you adopt the now overly familiar position in the stirrups.

A speculum is then inserted (without lubricant as this can affect the catheter) to visualise the cervix. When the doctor is happy that they can visualise the cervix, the ultrasound probe is placed above the uterus. The doctor then tells the embryologist she is ready for the catheter, which is passed through a hatch. I was able to watch on the screen as my little embryo was placed into my uterus in a flash of white. As I watched this magical moment, I gripped my good luck elephant that I had brought with me. The catheter is then returned to the embryologist to ensure that the transfer occurred, which takes about three or four minutes. My bladder was starting to give out at this stage, I was so full. I took the opportunity to ask if I could get a picture of the embryo for my journal and was told this would be no problem at all. The embryologist assured my doctor the catheter was clear, the speculum was removed and I was at last allowed to pee. When I had passed urine and gotten dressed, the nurse showed me the embryo on the computer and let me take pictures, she also told me she had frozen the image on the screen of the white flash and let me take pictures of that as well. An act of kindness that meant so much. I started my progesterone injections that day (I'd already started the progesterone vaginal gel a few days prior) and continued all other meds.

The next two weeks flew by, maybe because it was the run up to Christmas or maybe it was excitement. I had told myself at the start of this journey that I was going to enjoy the TWW. I did this; I enjoyed thinking I was pregnant. I did have heartburn, extremely sore breasts and for a few days I was very sensitive to smells. My beta HCG blood test was scheduled for the 30th December and I was told that I could do a home pregnancy test on the 28th December. I tested a couple of days early, after work.

It was negative and my world fell apart. I was working the next day so I didn't test that morning but I was keeping a little bit of hope alive that it was just too early, even though I knew in my heart that it wasn't a false negative. On the morning of the 28th December my world crumbled, I got up early and did two tests – both were negative. To make this day even worse, I was starting on a new ward that was opening the following week so I was there with my new CNM colleague, just the two of us. I wasn't even surrounded by people I knew and were my friends. I cried any time I was on my own that day, and for weeks after.

My family were so supportive and even though I knew I wasn't the only person this happened to, it felt like I was. My blood test confirmed what the home tests had shown. I asked that I be scheduled as soon as possible for my next FET because, although I was and still am devastated by the fail, I really want to succeed and it felt right for me to try again. I had such hopes, dreams and plans for the future for this baby and our life together. I would think I was ok and then I'd cry again without even thinking about it. I felt like my body had killed the embryo and that I had done something to cause this to happen. I met a friend of mine who had undergone IVF two years ago and her first cycle had also failed. She reassured me that she had felt the exact same and that what I was feeling was completely normal. She now has twin girls and is an inspiration.

I decided after my failed FET to try and lose weight, as I feel it'll improve my chances of a successful transfer. I have since brought my BMI down from 39 to 32.

In January 2021, I had my planning appointment with my doctor. The plan was to take the same meds as the December cycle and I'd have progesterone levels done the day of transfer and day of my beta HCG. I started acupuncture before my cycle began (which I am still thoroughly enjoying). My FET was booked for March 2021. Unfortunately, at my first scan my lining was only 4mm. I was devastated to say the least but determined not to give up. I began drinking 500mls of beetroot juice a day, increased my acupuncture to twice a week and began using my parents' treadmill every day. It all worked a little and my lining increased to 5.2mm in six days – the most growth I've had, but sadly still not good enough and again, my cycle was cancelled.

I spoke to my nurse at length at my last scan appointment and told her I felt the fact I'd been scheduled with my pill and not Provera® (as I had with the previous cycle) may have affected the lining, as the cancelled October cycle was also scheduled with Dianette®. She assured me she'd ask about this and I was both surprised and delighted when she rang back and told me that my doctor had agreed regarding the pill. I was to stop my meds and start Provera® the next day – I could go straight into another cycle!

My next FET is scheduled for the end of April 2021. I have continued acupuncture, beetroot juice, exercise and heat in the hope it'll all help. This will be my fifth cycle in nine months. I am physically, emotionally and mentally exhausted but I'll keep going until I have my baby or babies in my arms (they will transfer two embryos this time to increase my chance of success). I really could not have done this without the support of my family and friends. I haven't attended a clinic or acupuncture appointment on my own, there has always been at least one member of my family with me – even if that meant sitting in the car! I remain hopeful that this cycle is the one that makes me a mammy.

Connect with me on Instagram: @irishsmbcjourney

Chosen charity

My charity is Adapt Domestic Abuse Services: adaptservices.ie

They support women and children affected by domestic abuse, by providing emergency accommodation and outreach services (such as a helpline, support group and educational opportunities).

Erin and Nick

Following an infertility journey and IUI, Erin and Nick had twins in 2011. Six years later, they began a second journey for a sibling – one that led to IVF and seven transfers. They talk about their experience with an embryo reduction, multiple failed cycles, miscarriage and welcoming their rainbow baby.

Erin

Nick and I got married when I was 25. We knew we wanted kids and while we thought we would wait a couple of years, the summer of 2010 brought the baby itch. We started trying. I came off the pill and I wasn't getting a period. Being the instant gratification personality that I am, I booked an appointment with my obstetrician after a couple of months had gone by. I sat there, waiting for her to come in, and while this should have been an exciting moment in my life, it was absolutely terrifying, and little did I know what lay ahead. She explained to me that I didn't seem to ovulate on my own, in which case I would need fertility treatments to conceive a child. I was shocked. I didn't know anyone who'd had to do this, let alone at 26! So, she referred me to a specialist and we made an appointment.

I remember sitting in that waiting room for the first time. I felt embarrassed. I felt like I didn't belong there. I thought fertility treatments were only for older women, not me. But there we were, waiting to see what we needed to do.

The RE (reproductive endocrinologist) we met with suggested we first try an IUI, with the help of fertility drugs to stimulate my ovaries. Apparently, I had A LOT of follicles, but they weren't maturing and therefore not releasing. So, we started off with Clomid® – a drug to help stimulate your ovaries. That didn't work, so we moved on to a more invasive method of injecting my stomach every day and night with Menopur®. This would hopefully help the follicles grow and mature, and then with another injection, a few would release.

Sure enough, this method worked. We did what's called our 'trigger shot' and my follicles were on their way to being released. We came into the clinic for them to inseminate me with Nick's sperm, using a long syringe, and there we were – effectively pregnant until proven otherwise. I remember laying on the exam table for 20 minutes after they inseminated me, thinking how I would NEVER want to tell anyone about this. I already felt bad enough making Nick deal with it so there was no way I would ever be sharing the experience.

Two weeks later, I got my blood drawn to see if the IUI had worked. I have a very bad relationship with pregnancy tests, as up until then I had gotten so many negatives. I used to pee on the sticks three or four times in a row, thinking I must have done it wrong. This time, I just waited for that blood test. I didn't want them to call me, since Nick was at work, so I made them call him. I stayed in our apartment all day, pacing, not being able to think about anything else. And then suddenly Nick came barging in, with a huge grin! He picked me up and said, 'We are pregnant!'. Now that I felt safe, I called the doctor and they informed me that my first beta reading was at 1500. That is VERY high; they said it could possibly mean multiples but we would wait for the first ultrasound in a few weeks.

I bled A LOT the day before my ultrasound. The nurse said to just lay low but not to worry, it was normal. Obviously, I couldn't sleep that night. We went into the clinic and had our first ultrasound. With my legs wide open and my heart pounding fast, worried we had miscarried, the nurse looked up and said, 'Congratulations, you are having TRIPLETS!'. We were in shock, so thankful we were all ok, but triplets??? Immediately following the ultrasound, we were called into the doctor's office to discuss. He told us that I would be at high risk, meaning my own life would be at risk, along with the babies' lives, if we decided to carry all three. He said we should consider a reduction and that's what he would recommend: 'There is a clinic in LA you can go to, you just have to do this before 9 weeks'. Our hearts sank. How on earth could we make this decision? Yet, how would I survive mentally, worrying that our lives were at risk if we moved forward with three? We knew what we had to do and it was the most traumatic decision of our lives. I was 26 and Nick was 31.

We drove to LA and we stayed in a little hotel close to the clinic, as we had to be there first thing in the morning. We went in and the physician told us she would be aborting the embryo that was the easiest to get to. We didn't know the genders or anything of that sort, we didn't know if any of them were normal embryos or not, we just shook our heads and said 'ok'. I closed my eyes most of the time, I didn't want to watch. She said I would bleed out the remains and to take it easy for a couple of weeks. We were very quiet on the way home. We didn't tell anyone for years.

As hard as that was, I knew, and still know, we made the right choice. I carried my twin girls to term and birthed them vaginally! They were both perfectly healthy, except one of the girls, Eliana, was tiny since her umbilical cord was very thin. She needed more nutrients to get a little fatter so she stayed in the NICU for 11 days. Those were some of the hardest days of my life. I felt so guilty bringing one baby home and not the other. I was exhausted from being a new mom and driving to and from the NICU daily to feed and be with the other twin. But we did it. She came home after 11 days and has been the strongest, spunkiest child since.

In the months following, we found out I had a hernia from the pregnancy and that my stomach muscles had torn. We decided I needed to have that fixed so my back would stop hurting and I could regain my strength. I had Diastasis Recti surgery and hernia repair surgery in December 2011 – six months after the twins were born. I don't remember much, as they say you forget trauma, but I wasn't allowed to pick up the babies for six weeks. Thankfully, I had stored enough milk (since I was producing 22oz every three hours) to last them for an additional three months post-surgery.

Life went on. We were beyond grateful for our girls. But then they turned 6, and we knew we had to try for another baby. We stayed hopeful and tried on our own during the summer of 2017, and sure enough ended up back at the fertility clinic for help. This time, we would be jumping into IVF right away. I was elated. I thought ok, IVF meant I would be pregnant in four months! I would get to choose the gender and we would have this baby by the end of the coming summer. I was very wrong.

We paid for the first round. Unfortunately, here in California, insurance doesn't cover fertility treatments. So almost $30,000 per round (meaning egg retrieval to transfer) was what we had to pay up front. Forms were signed and we were on our way. We had our first egg retrieval and they collected eight eggs. Only three made it to full embryos and after sending them to get PGS tested, we only ended up with one normal embryo. But we only needed one, right? So, hopeful and honestly naïve, we transferred our one embryo in December

2017. This transfer failed. We were back at square one, devastated and in shock.

We tried again. Signed the forms, paid up front and went through another retrieval and transfer. We had the same results. We transferred one embryo, along with another one that was not normal but could potentially grow to be (termed a mosaic embryo) and they too failed. I didn't understand. I felt like I had all the pregnancy symptoms. But that's the thing with IVF, you are on so many hormones and fertility drugs that your body almost mimics pregnancy symptoms. It was such a mind game. I started to feel depressed. I felt so guilty that we had spent so much money and I had spent so much time going back and forth to the doctor, doing shots, bloodwork, and exams for nothing. I had taken so much time away from my twins (or so it felt like I had) and I couldn't handle that guilt.

After trying an IUI, and having it fail, we decided to take a break. We needed a break financially, mentally and I needed it physically. We were disconnected as a couple and my mind couldn't focus on anything other than IVF. We took the summer off to cleanse my body. I started acupuncture treatments regularly to help with fertility and I trained to become a yoga teacher. We travelled, and you better believe I was as present as I could be with my girls.

September 2018 came quick; we switched clinics because we weren't happy with our old one and tried for our third egg retrieval and third transfer. This time, we decided not to test our embryos. We had three and thought, due to the controversy of testing, we would take our chances. We were pregnant! It worked! I remember crying in my closet on the floor, so many tears of joy, of relief and shock. We didn't tell the girls right away and waited until six weeks to tell them, once we saw a heartbeat. They were so excited, they cried and we could not stop talking about that baby.

A couple of weeks later, it was time for me to 'graduate' from my fertility clinic and onto the OB: 'I'm sorry Erin, but the baby has stopped growing'. My world collapsed. We had miscarried. I remember holding on to Nick's shirt so tightly as he held me up so I wouldn't fall out of the bed. I couldn't even pull my pants up, how would I continue about my day? How would I tell the girls? But we did. They sobbed as we had to explain that the baby had died in my tummy. The guilt ate me alive.

I bled for about three months straight. I was told to take misoprostol, which is a pill to induce miscarriage. I was asked to catch any tissue that came out of me and save it for testing. I had to do this twice. The second time I took the pill, I bled through four sets of pyjamas and my bed sheets. I couldn't walk the next morning as I had lost so much blood. The bleeding continued, not as severe, but for three months, until finally the doctor discovered more tissue in my uterus. Yes, from the miscarriage. I had to have a D&C (a dilation and curettage, to remove the tissue). I couldn't believe it. I was so angry that this went on for so long because I couldn't move on. But I went into surgery and felt a sense of relief when it was done.

The tissue didn't show much, in fact, we don't really know why I miscarried, the doctors just assumed the embryo was abnormal. We tested the remaining two embryos because I wasn't about to have another miscarriage if I could help it. One came back normal, so we transferred that one and it failed.

I wasn't sure if I could keep going. We were now two years in – three retrievals, four transfers and a miscarriage in. But Nick encouraged me, he knows me too well. He said, 'I think you've got it in you to do one more retrieval'. So, we did. And we got three PGS normal embryos, the most ever! We transferred one in August in such high hopes, and it failed. I was miserable, and so confused. I had a pelvic MRI done and a biopsy on my uterus, and they found some inflammation and something called adenomyosis (a condition where the inner lining of the uterus breaks through the muscle wall of the uterus). I was on medication for that for three months. This killed me as it meant more waiting. December 2019 rolled around and it was time to transfer again. I mean, it should work now right? We 'fixed' my uterus!

Another failed transfer. I had one embryo left. I didn't even know if I could go through the transfer process again – the heartache of another loss and the physical and emotional pain of the process. I knew something had to change. I became my own advocate. I asked to speak to another doctor in the same clinic. I liked him and we connected so I asked to switch. I learnt that this was MY journey. I needed to be happy and confident in my process and having the right doctor was a huge part of it.

I also told him I wanted my uterine lining to be thicker. In the past, the doctors had always insisted on it being 7-8mm for transfer, but this time I said no. I said I wanted it to be at least 9.5mm. I checked my vitamin D levels, rechecked my thyroid and we were on our way to our seventh transfer. I felt the most positive and confident (and informed) as I had ever felt in the past. I knew this would work… And here I am, holding my rainbow baby, who is now 4 months old.

IVF was a roller coaster. A mind game to say the least. It almost broke me, it hurt my marriage at times and it took over my life for three years. But it also made me stronger; it made my marriage the strongest it has ever been. It made my little family closer. It helped my girls grow and become more compassionate. It made me humble and patient. But most of all, it made me into who I am today. I wouldn't wish this journey upon anyone but I also know had I not gone through it, I wouldn't be where I am today. Not only holding my little girl, that third baby I knew was meant to be ours one day, but it led me to growing into my own skin. To feeling powerful, stronger than ever and it has made me realise how incredibly strong I am, and I only hope that my girls will see that one day. Life is crazy. It's so unpredictable and I truly believe that the strongest ones, the warriors, go through all this because they are capable of coming out the other end.

Connect with me on Instagram:
@mybeautifulblunder

Chosen charity

Our charity is The Broken Brown Egg:
thebrokenbrownegg.org

They seek to empower, inform, and advocate for those questioning or experiencing the impact of infertility, with an emphasis on the Black experience of it.

Nadine and Guillaume

They have been TTC for four years, with two
IVF cycles and five transfers, resulting in one ectopic
pregnancy and a thoracic endometriosis diagnosis.
They talk about their fertility struggles with chronic
illness, a low ovarian reserve, and the ongoing journey
to having their rainbow baby.

Nadine

Endometriosis has dominated aspects of my life for more years than I care to remember. As a teenager, I spent my periods in excruciating pain, bedbound for up to seven days, constipated, bloated and nauseous. It took five years to be diagnosed by a private hospital. Thanks to my dad, I finally had a name for this pain. He demanded that my GP refer me to a gynaecologist. Why did it take so long? Why wasn't I listened to sooner? By the time I had my diagnostic laparoscopy, I already knew that I had endometriosis. But hearing that it was stage four and there was no cure, as well as being too young to have it removed, was disheartening.

I spent the next five years on the pill, taking it back-to-back until my body couldn't cope any more. At twenty-five years old, I was having a period and realised I couldn't get out of bed. At hospital, various teams struggled to manage and explain my symptoms. Endometriosis caused my lung to collapse and bowel obstruction. I had over a litre of fluid drained from my chest, before undergoing an emergency laparotomy. I remember waking up and being informed that I had a stoma and colostomy bag. I was put on Zoladex® injections and referred to an endometriosis centre. It was here that I learned endometriosis symptoms could disappear if I had a baby and that IVF would be the best option. At the time, I wasn't in a relationship where I wanted to consider it. Dealing with my colostomy and the side effects of being put into a menopausal state was enough.

In 2017, my partner and I embarked on our IVF journey. We were eligible for NHS funded treatment and our GP practice told us to choose a clinic. I didn't fully understand the process or know anyone who had gone through it. I opted for a hospital that had a good reputation overall and was easy to travel to. Sadly, in the January, my partner's father suddenly passed away. We were still grieving and just going through the motions of fertility treatment. It was a difficult time, but we felt it was best to proceed, in the hope that we could bring a new life in to the world.

It was strange having to inject myself every day. I was on a short protocol and I remember feeling quite tired after work and getting anxious at the idea of putting hormones into my body. With all the scar tissue in my abdomen, it often made the process quite painful. I would get calls at work from the embryology team with updates. Eighteen eggs were collected, thirteen fertilised and eight were frozen, with one fresh blastocyst transferred back to me. The stims took their toll on my body and the transfer was incredibly distressing. At home, I started bleeding before I took the pregnancy test. A few days later, the test was a BFN. I was then taken to A&E and diagnosed with OHSS. Some of the symptoms of this included sharp pains in my thighs, nausea, difficulty passing urine, and intense abdominal pain.

It took us a while to process the IVF experience. We took some time away from trying to conceive and focused on travelling, and spending quality time with family and friends. We married in 2018 and bought our first home together. This was the year we did our first frozen embryo transfer (FET). Mentally, we felt like we were in a much better place. I was a lot calmer as I knew my ovaries did not have to be stimulated. Transfer day came and went. On test day, I got up early to take the pregnancy test and took a photo of the result to send to my husband on WhatsApp before getting back into bed. Once he woke up, he asked me if I had tested and I casually mentioned I had sent him the result, which was... positive!! We were over the moon! It was truly the happiest moment of our lives. We allowed ourselves to dream and imagine being a family of three. Two embryos had been transferred so we didn't know if it would be twins. We kept seeing twins everywhere in the shops and just felt so full in our hearts that good news was coming our way and our lives would change forever.

On the day of our first scan, the last thing I looked at before we left home was the double-sided information sheet from the clinic in relation to test day and next steps if it was positive. It said at the bottom of the document that even if it is positive, it could result in an ectopic pregnancy. For some reason, this stuck with me and I just wanted to be extra cautious so tried to hold my breath until the scan. I had ordered my 'baby on board' badge, which had arrived a couple of days earlier, and I wore it for the first time on the tube.

Once we got to the station, I just sensed that something might not be right. I started to feel very anxious. We waited in the clinic for our names to be called for what felt like a very long time. The nurse started the scan but within seconds, she looked concerned because she couldn't see the fetus. I tried to keep calm as she moved us to another room with better equipment. Before I knew it, there were four or five medical professionals in the room, all looking alarmed and talking amongst themselves.

The consultant looked at me and broke the news that

it was ectopic. My husband did not know what it was, so they quickly explained that the baby was in my fallopian tube, and they insisted we make our way straight to their sister hospital to have the pregnancy surgically removed. I was in shock. My husband was heartbroken. Inside, I just wanted to scream and cry out. But I felt I had to keep calm so the surgeons could do what they needed to. My parents visited me at the hospital that night. And once they all left, I took a few moments to say goodbye to the baby I would never meet.

The next morning, I waited to be seen by a senior consultant, who seemed very concerned that there was a heartbeat. I was told I would lose my right fallopian tube and possibly the ovary too. I broke down in tears and begged them to let me keep my ovary as I did not have any children. In my notes it said the findings were highly suggestive of interstitial ectopic pregnancy. Apparently, these count for up to 6% of ectopic pregnancies and carry a higher risk of a life-threatening haemorrhage. The surgery took hours because of my extensive endometriosis. Fortunately, they called on another surgeon with more experience to ensure the ovary stayed intact.

Once I was discharged, I remember being back home and in the early hours of the morning, I touched my stomach and realised I was bleeding. One of the wound sites was not healing. My husband, mum and I spent just under twenty-four hours at hospital. Finally, they used stitches to stop the bleed and sent me home again. Weeks went by and we got the keys to our first home. Neither of us discussed it but the room we thought would be the baby's room was not really used. It just didn't feel the same.

As we got into 2019, and each year after, friends had

their first babies and announced their pregnancy news. Time went by and we became stronger and able to be genuinely happy for others as we continued our fertility journey. That year, I did two FETs (one with one embryo and another with two embryos). They both resulted in BFN. To complicate things further, I was experiencing breathing problems and a heaviness on my chest. In the summer, I had a pleural effusion, which caused a litre of fluid to build on my lung. At the end of the year, in December, I had surgery for a haemothorax, and an excellent team operated on my right lung and diaphragm. I was on the ward for twelve days and allowed to go home on Christmas Eve, which was the best present ever!

As 2020 approached, we felt hopeful and met with a new fertility clinic. My initial tests were delayed because of the pandemic. Once the results came in, we were told that I was too high risk because I am a BAME woman with a history of endometriosis, adenomyosis and thoracic endometriosis. They told me DEIVF (donor egg IVF) was my best option. I did not know much about DEIVF and tried to still have a positive mindset, despite feeling that my body was useless.

We were still determined to do an FET that year, so went back to the NHS as private patients and used two frozen embryos. My body did not respond to the medication initially, so I had to abandon treatment and do an HSG. The results came back normal and I was given my usual drugs, plus oestrogen gel. The transfer was traumatic, and my uterus was tilted so they struggled to get the embryos in the right place. Despite them being really good quality embryos, on test day it was another BFN. I called my mum and cried on the phone hysterically because I was starting to lose hope.

We had attended an open day at another clinic in

2019 and were impressed with them. I researched one of their consultants, who had expertise in implantation. After numerous tests and a consultation, they were happy to take us on as patients in 2021. I was told my AMH had reduced to a third of what it was in 2017 because of my endometriosis, which meant that my stims had to be much higher than before. There was some adenomyosis in my uterus, but it was under control. In my right ovary was a 3cm cyst.

The experience so far has been very positive. All the staff are lovely and know me by name. I felt like the clinic was my second home in the lead up to the egg collection. Including the baseline scan, I had six scans and was always given clear information about the quality of my eggs. The left ovary was high up and stuck behind the bowel, therefore, only the right ovary was used to collect follicles, but this was the one that had a greater number. I almost burst into tears when they told me nine eggs had been collected. Throughout the whole experience, I had been very cautious and tried not to get my hopes up because of what the other clinic had said. I got daily updates from the clinic and four fertilised normally, two of them became high grade embryos suitable for freezing. I couldn't help comparing this with the nine embryos I had with the NHS cycle. But then my husband reminded me that my ovarian reserve was higher then and those embryos didn't result in a baby.

Unfortunately, the day after egg collection, I felt quite unwell. It was difficult to pass urine and I could not walk upright. I went to A&E, where they diagnosed me with OHSS (again), a distended abdomen and they discovered the cyst in my ovary was bleeding. I am so grateful to the NHS for taking such good care of me during my short stay in hospital whilst we are in a pandemic. I am also immensely grateful to the thoracic team who helped me have a better quality of life and be physically fit enough to continue fertility treatment.

My husband, family, friends, and the online community have been my rock since the pandemic. Having a safe space to express my joys and vulnerabilities means the world to me. I thank everyone for their thoughts and prayers. I trust in God and know that one day, somehow or another, I will become a parent. I have two attempts with these new frozen embryos and one still with the NHS. I am prepared to do one more egg collection before considering DEIVF. And... a very lovely person has just offered to be a surrogate! I am tearful writing this because she has no idea what a generous offer that is. Surrogacy has always been something we were open to because of implantation failure, but we never thought we would find such a selfless person willing to gift this to us. For my husband and I, we are grateful to have come this far and are excited for the future.

Thank you for reading and please feel free to connect with me on Instagram:
@endometriosisandme1

Chosen charity

Our charity is The Ectopic Pregnancy Trust:
ectopic.org.uk

The trust believes the deaths and trauma associated with ectopic pregnancy should be prevented or minimised, and they seek to support women and their families through this difficult period in their lives.

Pandora and James

After being diagnosed with a varicocele, they TTC for nine months before seeking help. Learning they had severe male factor infertility, they pursued ICSI via IVF. Three transfers later, they are pregnant with their baby boy. They talk about their experience with an ectopic pregnancy, a chemical pregnancy and experiencing pregnancy after IVF and loss.

Pandora

The story of how James and I met is quite unique. I was travelling in Australia from the UK and had only arrived two weeks prior. It was a Monday night and my friends had dragged me to a dodgy bar in Sydney. As soon as I saw him, I knew I liked him. He looked very intense and quite scary. I was the one to approach him. I think this took him by surprise and he wasn't used to girls being quite as forward as I was. I asked him so many questions about his beliefs and views on life, he must have thought I was completely insane but I guess he liked it, as he asked for my number and took me out three days later.

After dating only around a month, we were lying in bed when I asked him if he knew about the lump in one of his testicles. Not really a conversation I have had before. We started to get very concerned and booked an ultrasound the following day. The technician said straight away: 'Okay, it's not cancer so you can relax. It looks like a varicocele (an enlargement of the veins within the scrotum) and just so you know, this can affect sperm quality'. I remember thinking, 'Well, that's a little concerning'. We both had already discussed wanting children later in life.

When we went to the doctor for the results, we asked him about this and he said, 'There's no scientific evidence that a varicocele can affect male fertility, you should be fine'. Looking back, I wish I had done more research and not taken what this doctor said to be true.

We lived in Australia for a year and then went back to live in England for three years. Six years after the night we met, we got married. Our wedding was a beautiful overseas wedding in Bali. Being from opposite sides of the world, it was the first time our families had met. We actually started trying for a baby around three months before the wedding, hoping not to show on the day... how naïve.

Every month I would think 'this is it', but of course, every test was negative and we knew deep down something was wrong. We kept trying for another six months then went to get a semen analysis. The GP was so reluctant to do the test for us. He said we should keep trying for a year before any tests, but I said no... 'We want the test now' and I am so glad I did. The results were shocking. James had 2 million sperm count per mil, when the norm is 15-39 million. His motility was extremely low too, with 80% completely non-progressive – meaning they were not even moving. The doctor said, 'With results like this you need to see a specialist'. I wanted to laugh in his face for doubting we needed the test in the first place but the tears held me back. I have wanted to be a mum since I was six years old. I was obsessed with being mummy to my many dolls and pets growing up and I'd waited to find the perfect guy to share the experience with. Now I had found him, we were faced with this.

I wasn't going to wait around for an appointment, so I started calling male factor infertility specialists that day and found one that could see us in two weeks' time. I remember this time in my life being quite dark. I was so consumed by thoughts that we wouldn't be able to have a baby. I have read that other women think IVF is an instant solution and feel it will work first time – I didn't have this view. We headed to the clinic with open minds. The doctor wanted to do his own tests and check me out too. I had an internal scan and a series of blood tests, which all came back with no surprises. I was so relieved, as for some reason, I'd just assumed they would find more issues. James' test results were even worse than the first. They said to conceive naturally we had a 0.02% chance and we needed to pursue IVF. I said, 'Okay, when?'. He said we could start next time I got my period. I waited anxiously to start my injections.

This is when I set up a different Instagram page. I wanted somewhere to vent and express my emotions and I thought this could help – I never in a million years realised the amazing community I was walking in to. I connected with other girls going through the same process and asked hundreds of questions. It was amazing to have so much knowledge and advice at the tip of my fingers. Unlike other bloggers and 'Instagram socialites' I had come across, these ladies always replied with words of wisdom and kindness. One thing I will say to anyone reading this about to start treatment: make an Instagram page. You can keep it anonymous if that works for you, but just to connect with other people going through the same thing. It's a support system like no other. Family and friends try their best to be there for you but unless they have undertaken fertility treatments, they will say the wrong things at times. They won't understand how you are feeling and it can all be so lonely.

The injections themselves were quite simple. I found myself looking forward to them each night – it meant we were moving forward. I stimmed for 11 days, which I believe is a fairly normal, short protocol. By day 11, I was ready for my egg retrieval, if not slightly nervous. I'd never had any surgeries in the past or been

367

put under local anaesthetic. I tried to be as healthy as possible while stimming and stuck to fresh foods and no processed or high sugar meals. I am usually a pretty healthy person and being brought up by a Hippy mum, I've always lived a pretty low toxic lifestyle. I know this is a big movement in the fertility world, so I felt like I was already kind of ahead of the game.

The procedure went smoothly and I remember waking up and looking down at my hand, which had a big number 12 written on the palm of my hand. 12 eggs! I remember being so obsessed with numbers at this point. I would frantically research how many eggs were normal to retrieve and look at other women's fertility accounts to see how many they'd gotten. I think the fact I was coming down from all the hormones, more bloated than I had ever been in my life, and recovering from surgery made me so emotional. The next day, I received a call from the lab saying nine of the eggs were mature. I felt my numbers were diminishing quickly but was reminded by other ladies that it really only takes one great egg to make a baby. Even knowing that, every time the phone rang my heart would stop beating and I would hold my breath to hear the new number.

We were so lucky; we ended up with five embryos on transfer day. They transferred my best quality embryo and told me we had a 60% chance of success. I was full of hope and excitement. The two-week wait is everything I thought it would be: a full rollercoaster of emotions. One day you think, 'Yep, this is it. I'm pregnant', the next day you're sure it hasn't worked. I went back and forth constantly until day six, when I decided enough was enough and I had to take a test. I took a cheap one I had in my bathroom (biggest mistake ever) and it was a stark white negative. It was night time too, even though I knew the best time to take it was first thing in the morning. That was it, dreams crushed.

The next day was day seven and also Valentine's day. I woke up early and decided to test again. I took a First Response™ test this time (this is now the only test I will use in future). This one was positive! I couldn't believe it. I stared at it for a good three minutes before running out to my husband. We were completely over the moon. It had worked first time, and on Valentine's day too – we felt so lucky.

Three days later, blissfully unaware of any issues, I was at work, thinking about how I was pregnant and feeling pretty smug. I went to the bathroom, looked down and saw my knickers were full of blood! I started crying immediately (looking back, I was so uneducated on anything pregnancy related and this could've been completely normal). I called my clinic and asked what I should do. My nurse said I shouldn't rely on home pregnancy tests as these can be so inaccurate. I thought, 'Well, four tests can't be wrong'. I had taken one a day since the positive to see my lines progress and get darker. She said it could be okay and she would move my blood test to day 10 (the following day). When they called me with the results, she said, 'All those sneaky tests you've been taking are right, you are pregnant!'. I asked what my HCG was and she said 88, which is good. I could breathe again. We repeated the blood test and my numbers doubled accordingly. All signs pointed to a healthy pregnancy.

The bleeding subsided for two weeks and we even managed to take a little trip to Perth. Being pregnant made me feel so lucky. I was happy every day; it was all I had ever wanted. When we got back from our trip, I woke up in the night with terrible cramps. I called the out of hours clinic number and they said if there was no bleeding then it didn't sound like a miscarriage. I woke in the morning and the cramping had gone, so I thought maybe it was just normal in early pregnancy – I made excuses for every sign something was wrong. That afternoon, I stood up to walk our dog, Mavis, and blood gushed out of me. A lot of blood. I fell to the floor in tears and James put me in the car and drove me to the emergency room. I still remember his exact words when we got there: 'My wife is having a miscarriage'. I thought this can't be happening. Everything had gone to plan.

The treatment I received at the emergency room was horrendous. I was taken in, put in a hospital gown and the nurse asked me how far along I was. I told her I was six weeks pregnant and she said, 'Well, at least it's early on'. This made me so angry. I explained that we'd undergone IVF treatment to get here and that this pregnancy was extremely wanted. In losing a child there are no 'at least's! She said, 'Why are you doing IVF when you're so young?' – I instantly knew this woman was uneducated and not to listen to any of her remarks.

She took me to a bed and said she would need to take some blood. Having had hundreds of blood tests for treatment, I wasn't too worried. This was the worst blood test I've ever had though – she couldn't get my vein for around 20 minutes and ended up bruising both of my arms. She then dropped the vile of blood all over my gown. I sat there, in the emergency room, covered in blood, crying my heart out. We waited for three hours and then were told she hadn't taken enough blood (or as she put it, they had 'lost one on the way') and would need to send some more. Another three hours later, we got the results and my HCG was now 736.

This was a lot lower than we expected but still within range of a normal pregnancy.

Ten hours after we arrived, the doctor finally came to speak to us. I had a million questions. He couldn't confirm a miscarriage as it was too early for a scan (it was not) but because the bleeding had now stopped, he didn't think I'd lost the baby. I asked if it could be bleeding from the progesterone pessaries I was using and he told me I shouldn't be taking progesterone. I decided to just get out of the hospital and call my clinic. They had no experience with IVF or what the protocols were. My clinic told me to come in on Monday for a repeat blood test. I was left for the rest of the weekend wondering what was happening to my baby, and if there was even a baby in there anymore.

Two days later, I headed into my clinic for another blood test. I'd been frantically Googling everything I could think of and kept seeing 'ectopic pregnancy' appear. The nurse taking my blood asked me how I was doing and I told her what had happened over the weekend. I asked her if maybe this could point to an ectopic pregnancy and she told me that if it was ectopic, I'd be in so much pain I wouldn't be able to walk – which is completely untrue. I thought, 'Okay I'm not in any pain at all now so it can't be that'. My results came back as 1050 and the nurse said things were still looking alright, just on the low side. The main thing was that the number was increasing. She booked me in for my first ultrasound at eight weeks pregnant.

The day of my first ultrasound came and this day is by far the worst day of my life to date. I was at work, nervous but excited to finally see my baby and hear that little heartbeat. I said to my work colleague, 'I'll be back in about an hour'… I ended up coming back four weeks later. I got to the clinic and told my doctor I was a little nervous because of the bleeding and he explained how that can be totally normal in a healthy pregnancy. The ultrasound nurse got me up on the bed and they started an internal ultrasound. I remember her moving Wanda (the probe) around a lot, searching, and I instantly knew it was bad news. I squeezed James' hand and he whispered, 'It's okay'. She called my doctor in and I said, 'It's bad, isn't it?', she replied, 'No, I just get everything ready for him'. He came in, looked at the screen and said, 'Oh yeah, this doesn't look good'. I burst into tears. I know there is no good way of telling someone this news, but I feel as a doctor who has probably seen this a very high number of times, he should've worked on his wording. He then said that it looked like I'd miscarried.

The rest of that visit was a blur. I was pretty hysterical and I know they took my blood again and told me they would be in touch, that I should go home and rest. I remember not only being heartbroken but also extremely scared of what was going to happen. Would I see the baby when I miscarried or had it already happened? I was so confused. Being eight weeks, I thought the baby was the size of a raspberry and I was scared I would be in a lot of pain.

When I got home, my doctor called me – this was strange as he'd never called me before, only the nurses. Even to tell me I was pregnant. He said that my HCG was still increasing and he just wanted to be certain it wasn't an ectopic pregnancy, so asked if I could go to a special ultrasound place the following day, which had better machines. I asked if he thought this was ectopic, as I hadn't had any pain to one side or shoulder pain, which I'd read were common symptoms. He said, 'No I don't, but I want to be certain'. I booked myself in and went back to bed to cry some more.

That night, I woke at around midnight with a weird sensation that kind of felt like I needed the bathroom but when I got there, I collapsed to the floor in agony. The worst pain I have ever felt in my life. My insides felt like they were ripping open. James ran into the bathroom and called an ambulance. As I waited on the floor, I thought, 'This is probably just a miscarriage and I am really weak, and they're going to think I'm stupid'. I told James to cancel the ambulance but he wouldn't, he thought this was bad. Thank god he didn't, because I could have died

The paramedics were wonderful. They were so kind and caring, and completely looked after me in every way they could. They said all the right things and didn't make me feel stupid or mad, like so many other people in this field had done so far. They said even if it was a 'normal miscarriage' (whatever that is), I was better to go to the hospital and get pain relief. They gave me morphine to get me up off the floor and drove me to the hospital. Again, I had another blood test... again, my levels were rising. The nurses in the emergency room rotated a lot. Every nurse asked me how far along I was – every time I told the story again, and every time my heart broke. Most of the nurses didn't really know what to say and would try and keep me positive, saying, 'You never know, maybe the last scan was wrong'. I didn't need this false hope. One nurse sat on the edge of my bed and told me how she had experienced a miscarriage a month ago. Tears filled her eyes and I hugged her. This is what I needed – someone to relate to, someone who understood. I waited for an ultrasound machine to become available and lay there, wishing that they'd made a mistake and they would see a flicker.

I ended up having three different doctors do ultrasounds for me. These were so painful as they would press on my abdomen, even for the internal ones. I chose to look away every time. I didn't want to see that same empty uterus I'd seen at my IVF clinic. Finally, the last doctor told me it was an ectopic pregnancy and that the baby was at the end of my left fallopian tube, right next to my ovary. She said my tube had ruptured and my abdomen was full of blood. I asked her if she would need to remove the ovary but she couldn't say for sure until she'd seen it in surgery. This filled me with panic. What if this had ruined my chances of ever being a biological mother? I couldn't believe this had happened after they'd put the embryo into my uterus – how had it gotten into my tube?

James had left for a really important meeting at work. It was the one day he'd said he wouldn't be available and of course, this was the day I needed major surgery. I called and explained what the doctor had said and told him to come back. I was filled with fear and heartache. But being really honest, I felt a little lighter too, knowing I wasn't insane. I had known deep down from the first bleed that it wasn't normal and I knew something bad was happening inside my body.

I stayed in hospital for three days in total. It was nice to have constant help and pain relief. I had a lot of bleeding after the surgery and they'd put in a drain to get the blood from my abdomen. The surgeon showed me pictures from the surgery afterwards. He showed me the lump in my tube and I could see the baby. I could see the features of their face. He said they never had a heartbeat and that's why it was so hard to pick up on an ultrasound. Seeing the pictures made it much more real and I felt some closure.

Once I no longer needed the morphine, it was time to go home. I lay in bed for three weeks, watching endless Disney movies and going in and out of a deep depression. I finally thought maybe it was time to get some help, so I reached out to one of my clinic's therapists for a session. At the time, I would say I didn't really find her very helpful and decided one session was enough. Looking back now, it's probably what got me out of bed and back to work.

Returning to normality was tricky after all of that. Having to tell people I was no longer pregnant was extremely difficult for me. To top it off, we were faced with COVID-19 and navigating through a global pandemic. I returned to work at the height of it all here in Australia, which was a good distraction for me because my work became extremely busy.

When my period returned six weeks after surgery, I threw myself into another cycle. This time, I wasn't excited or hopeful. I was scared. I knew that once you have experienced an ectopic pregnancy, you're more likely to experience another, so I was on edge the entire cycle.

Transfer day came and the doctor popped in another embryo, this one with a 59% chance of success. I asked what success meant? Technically, my last transfer was a success as I got a positive pregnancy test. But my doctor assured me success means a live birth. I tested on day seven – the same day as the last TWW. I saw that second line, only this time it was so faint I could barely make it out. I knew if it got darker the next day it was a good sign so I waited and tested again. These days now just blur into a mess in my mind. Initially, the tests got darker then lighter again, and I knew it was over. My beta came back at 6. A chemical pregnancy. The embryo had attempted to attach but it was not successful.

At this point, my shell had hardened and I was no longer positive for the future of having a baby. I wanted one more transfer and then I told myself I would take a break. This time, I anticipated the worst. The TWW actually flew by because I didn't want to test. I was too terrified. I decided to test on day eight this time. I took the test and left it in the bathroom while me and James talked about the outcome. I made my way over to look at the test and from the door, I saw two beautiful, dark lines. I screamed and burst into tears. It just felt so different. I didn't take another test this time, I waited for my blood test and my HCG was 510! Four days later, it was at 3415. Even though the numbers were high, I still pushed for an early scan. I wanted to be sure I wasn't going to lose my right tube too.

I couldn't sleep the night before my first ultrasound. My doctor's words played over and over in my head from the last time, 'this doesn't look good'. What if he said that again? What would I do? James couldn't come to the scan this time, due to Covid restrictions, so I would be completely alone.

Ten minutes before my appointment, my clinic called to reschedule the ultrasound as the doctor didn't work on Wednesdays. I lived an hour away at the time and this sent me over the edge. I was hormonal, tired and extremely anxious. I burst into tears at the reception and they took me into the doctor's room and gave him a call. He agreed to come in to see me in two hours so I waited there, alone with my thoughts. I was very appreciative that he was coming but again, terrified. When he got there, he said it was better to know now if anything was wrong and we should get started. I closed my eyes and hoped for the best. When I opened them, I could see a black spot – a gestational sac. He said this was good and meant chances were, it wasn't ectopic. He told me to come back in two weeks and that is when I saw my baby's heart beating for the first time.

The entire pregnancy has gone completely to plan. I experienced the worst morning sickness, but I was glad, as this killed my anxiety a little for the first trimester. Perfect ultrasounds every step of the way. A growing belly that I am in love with and just overall, an amazing pregnancy filled with all those fun symptoms. However, experiencing pregnancy after loss has not been easy. I have tried to get out of the mindset to expect bad news at every appointment but this has proven harder than I thought. Every ultrasound was riddled with fear and sleepless nights in the build-up. The further along I've gotten, the more confident I have become. I am currently thirty-three weeks along and eagerly anticipating my baby boy's arrival. I can't actually believe I'm here after everything that's happened. It really has made me appreciate every single part of pregnancy.

Although I have experienced such heartache and loss, I have also gained so much. I am part of a wonderful community of infertility warriors. I have gained crucial friends for life, that have given me support throughout this journey, who I now could not live without. It really is the worst club with the best members. I have had so many beautiful messages since sharing my story online, saying I have given women hope after loss and I hope by writing my story, I can bring someone else hope. Infertility is something that is not talked about enough.

Connect with me on Instagram: @ttcbabychevs

Chosen charity

Our charity is Resolve: resolve.org

Resolve: The National Infertility Association is dedicated to ensuring all people challenged in their family building journey reach resolution through being empowered by knowledge, supported by community, united by advocacy, and inspired to act.

Hannah

Hannah, 31, and her husband, 35, live in the UK and have been TTC for over two years, during which time Hannah was diagnosed with stage 3 endometriosis. They've undergone IVF with a private clinic, which sadly resulted in an early miscarriage. Hannah shares her infertility journey and the newfound resilience she's gained. She also gives reference to her mother, who suffered unexplained infertility and sought fertility treatment years prior to Hannah's own battles.

Hannah and her husband continue to pursue fertility treatment in their dream to become parents.

Hannah

Once upon a time, I thought getting pregnant was easy, and that intense and heavy periods were normal. Those were the times 'pre-infertility', where I was blissfully unaware of the challenges that I would begin to encounter in my late 20s and early 30s. I always knew that I wanted to be a mum, and when I met my now-husband I knew instantly that one day, when we felt ready to grow our family, we would make the most incredible parents. Our story however, has not been without its challenges, and I'd therefore like to share my experience in the hope that it provides some comfort to anyone else on their own infertility journey.

So here I sit, writing my story, after more than two years of trying to get pregnant, with a newfound empathy for so many other women out there who are still waiting for their first born. For those reading this, I wish to firstly acknowledge that you are not alone, you are enough, you are strong, and you CAN do this!

Long before my own battles began, my mum was one of the many women suffering with infertility. We are both part of 'the club'; we are 1 in 8. It's the worst club to be part of, but the community is full of wonderful and incredibly brave women, and without it I wouldn't be in a position to share my story. Before the days of social media (which is certainly a very accessible way to connect with each other) my parents, in their attempts to grow their family, suffered with 'unexplained infertility'. Fortunately, despite lots of investigations and years of trying, they eventually conceived me naturally, but to never be given a true reason why it took so long feels so incredibly unfair when all you want are answers.

During my parents' attempts to then try for a sibling for me, they had similar battles, and conceived via IUI. Tragically, my mum lost the baby at 18 weeks and whilst I don't remember too many details of that period in our lives as I was quite young, I will never forget or take for granted how difficult that must have been for my parents. Having now experienced a miscarriage myself, at a very early stage, I understand the pain, but to have it happen at such a late stage is just unimaginable.

My parents' story did however end happily, when they conceived my wonderful sister via IUI a year later. I am so deeply respectful and proud of my mum for her courage, and all that she experienced and endured both physically and emotionally during those times. She deserves a special reference in my story because she, along with my amazing friends and other members of my family, including my husband, have been my absolute rock. My mum has been the one person I can turn to who understands everything I'm feeling and she always knows the right words to say. I honestly couldn't imagine battling infertility without her and whilst it hurts me that we both are having to endure this pain, she gives me the motivation and hope to stay strong. One day, I can't wait to look at her, with a baby in my arms and say, 'I did it Mum, I can finally call myself a Mum'. I know she will read this so, 'thank you Mum, I love you to the moon and back'.

My infertility story began a few years after my husband and I got married, and after some incredible holidays and adventures together that I'll never forget. When nothing happened after the first six months of trying, I remember having a gut feeling that something was wrong. Despite feeling a bit 'silly' and 'negative' for having those thoughts, I just couldn't dismiss the concern. Perhaps because I knew what my mum had endured, I thought maybe I would have a similar experience. Even though at that stage, I had no actual reason to validate those concerns.

My gut feeling did, however, lead me to book a consultation with a gynaecologist for peace of mind. Ironically, we ended up seeing the very same gynaecologist who helped my mum conceive my sister via IUI. It felt comforting to know we would be in good hands and this expert could give my husband and I answers. If she could help my parents, of course she could help us. I also remember at the time, people I'd mentioned my fears to telling me to be patient and to stop thinking negatively and worrying. Whilst I am a very impatient person, and I respected the advice I received, I am so glad I listened to my gut and booked that appointment, or I wouldn't have got the answers I needed.

Fortunately, I was able to seek infertility investigations privately due to my employer's private healthcare, which was a blessing as it meant we didn't have to wait to be referred by our GP or wait for NHS funding (something we knew could have delayed matters). At this point, we'd only been trying for about seven months so we also knew the NHS would've made us wait at least a year before starting investigations. Despite being very anxious about the first consultation at the clinic, it was absolutely worth it and I would urge anyone who's in a similar position to trust your gut and make the first step to seeking answers.

The process for the investigations was extremely quick and efficient, and included carefully timed blood tests during my menstrual cycle, some internal ultrasounds to check my ovaries and uterus, and a semen analysis for my husband. The results all came back normal. Even my AMH level, which assesses your ovarian reserve, was in the 'good/normal' range and there were no concerns identified or reasons to explain why we weren't getting pregnant.

However, our gynaecologist did raise some concerns about my menstrual cycle – in particular, the fact that prior to each cycle, I get brown spotting a few days before a 'full flow'. I'd also told her that as a teenager I had incredibly painful periods, which had led to my GP putting me on the contraceptive pill to manage the symptoms, instead of investigating the cause. I'd just thought painful and heavy periods were normal, however the gynaecologist commented that spotting and painful and heavy periods can be a symptom of endometriosis. She told us that if we weren't able to conceive naturally in the following six months, I should have further investigations to determine if I had the condition, which can also cause infertility. This was the first time I'd ever heard the word 'endometriosis' and I'll be honest, I had absolutely no idea what it was – which seems pretty crazy when I was soon to learn that unfortunately, the condition affects 1 in 10 women and is incredibly common and debilitating for many.

We left the clinic, prepared to start using ovulation tests every month to identify my peak 'fertile window' and the best time to try to conceive naturally. I also remember instantly typing 'endometriosis' into Google, where I learnt that it's a chronic condition where tissue similar to the lining of the womb starts to grow in other places in the body, such as the ovaries and fallopian tubes, and it can affect women of any age. I quickly found out the worst part of the condition, alongside the many horrific symptoms, is that it's long term and incurable. There is currently no cure.

You can imagine my emotions as I started to discover more about it. Whilst I was comforted by the fact that I wasn't alone (given how common it is), nor is it life threatening, I did feel a sense of panic that there was a chance I could actually have this. Prior to the ongoing infertility investigations, I had fortunately never endured any serious illnesses. I'd never been in hospital for surgery or sickness, and generally I considered myself to be a healthy woman with no underlying health conditions. I soon realised, having read through the listed symptoms, that I didn't seem to have the same severity of symptoms as many other women endure, which made me feel extremely grateful. Apart from bad period pains causing some absence from school and work in my teenage years, I wouldn't say that the pain ruined or significantly impacted years of my life. I have so much respect for women who have to deal with the severe and debilitating symptoms daily and I only hope that one day there will be a cure – or a way to improve the lives of women who are so deeply affected by the condition.

Six months after our appointment with the gynaecologist, when the first reference to endometriosis was made, we still hadn't had any success conceiving naturally. I had never seen a positive pregnancy test and the monthly disappointment was becoming increasingly difficult to comprehend. Little did we know, at that point our journey was only beginning.

We went back to the clinic to discuss next steps to investigate and determine if I did have endometriosis. It was at this appointment I was told that the only way to diagnose endometriosis is via keyhole surgery, called a laparoscopy. I was told this would require me to have a general anaesthetic. Listening to our gynaecologist explain the details of the procedure made me feel really nervous, and quite frankly, sick. I had an overwhelming feeling of 'is this really happening to me?'. I remember her explaining that they'd need to make small incisions in my stomach and lower region in order to put cameras inside me to identify any signs of endometriosis and if it was discovered around my organs, and extractable, they would essentially remove it. This would only be temporary though, as the condition causes the endometriosis to grow back.

I remember leaving that appointment, getting in the car with my husband and just sobbing. My biggest fear was the general anaesthetic – worrying that I might not wake up. These fears were quickly settled by family and friends who'd had a general anaesthetic, and especially by my mum, who'd had the exact same procedure when she was my age. Speaking about my concerns really helped me overcome my fears, and I think it's only natural to have fears of the unknown. I allowed myself to have those feelings but made sure to try my hardest to apply a rational perspective, to help me not panic.

Soon after that appointment, I had the laparoscopy, and I can honestly say that the thought of it was far worse than the reality. It's highly likely that in my lifetime I will need further procedures, and having gone through it, I feel much more relaxed if that happens in the future. I had the comfort of my husband with me, and my mum, and we had a lovely private room which helped my nerves. I remember being so worried about the needle for the general anaesthetic that I'd researched and purchased (very expensive) numbing cream, which I'd generously applied to my hands and arms before arriving at the clinic, as I wasn't sure where the cannula would be inserted. I think the nurses must have thought I was crazy, but it gave me peace of mind and I didn't feel a thing when the needle went in! Since that time, I've had further general anaesthetics and I didn't bother with the numbing cream, so it really goes to show that the fear of the unknown is so powerful and once it's no longer the unknown, your fears are quickly diminished.

Immediately following the procedure, I remember waking up after a wonderfully deep sleep. The first thing I ate was a biscuit and it tasted incredible. It was so good that my husband proceeded to order 100 small packets for our house, which made me laugh so much when they were delivered as a surprise (I promise we didn't eat them all and enjoyed sharing them with family!). It's funny how you can create little memories around periods of sadness and difficulty in your life, and I'll treasure those moments that felt insignificant at the time. I'll also never forget our gynaecologist coming into our room shortly after I'd woken up and informing me that they'd found endometriosis, but they'd removed it and I was 'as good as new'.

I cried tears of relief and fear at the same time. I was so thankful to have an answer, unlike my mum who never got that with her unexplained infertility, but I felt a sense of dread, because now I knew that I had an incurable condition that caused infertility. I remember thinking, 'will I ever become a mum?'. Sadly, writing this now, I still ask myself that same question on a daily, or even hourly, basis. Unfortunately, there are just so many things in life that trigger those thoughts.

Our gynaecologist also informed us that women are at 'peak' fertility after a laparoscopy and she therefore advised that once we felt ready and I'd recovered from the procedure (which did leave me feeling very tender for a couple of weeks), we should try to conceive naturally. I remember searching online for 'success stories after a laparoscopy' and discovered several, which gave me so much positivity and hope for the months to follow.

The recovery wasn't too bad, and after the first four days of feeling rather tender and tired, I began to feel a bit more like myself. I was fortunate to have been signed off work for two weeks for the recovery and I would encourage anyone having this procedure to have at least a week off work just to heal, both physically and emotionally. I am so thankful for those two weeks off as I felt so well-rested as a result. I was eager and excited to try to conceive naturally with the hope that my body (or insides at least) were cleansed of this awful endometriosis. I was also feeling a sense of impatience because I knew the removal of the endometriosis was only temporary and it could grow back soon after.

My husband and I didn't waste any time and once I felt comfortable, I was back relying on ovulation sticks and my cycle tracking app to identify my fertile window. I also continued to search online forums for success stories after a laparoscopy and felt extremely positive when I found many stories of women conceiving as soon as a month or two after the procedure. I so wished to become one of those women, but sadly, it wasn't on the cards for me.

Three months after the procedure, and three months of failed attempts, we were back where it all began nearly a year prior, asking now to be referred for fertility treatment. At this point, the COVID-19 pandemic had hit the world and appointments were held virtually instead of face-to-face. During our virtual appointment, which was via a phone call, our gynaecologist informed us that my endometriosis had been diagnosed as stage 3 which, I'd later discover through yet more research, meant my condition was considered 'moderate', involving deep implants on my ovaries and pelvic lining. In short, it didn't feel like good news.

We were then told that as a result of the severity of the endometriosis, it meant our options for fertility treatment were somewhat restricted. We were told the success rates of trying to conceive via IUI were extremely low for those with stage 3 endometriosis. Therefore, we were recommended to start IVF in the first instance. I felt like I had a good understanding of IUI because of how my mum conceived my sister, and I knew it wasn't overly expensive compared to IVF. I didn't know much at all about IVF, other than there would be injections involved, which made me feel nervous.

It was at this appointment it felt as though our journey had taken a new turn and really intensified. Not only had we been told that IVF was our best chance, but that, because of Covid, there would likely be an impact on fertility treatment and we had to wait to see what would unfold over the following months. At this point, I remember thinking how the whole infertility journey is all about waiting and finding your inner patience, which for me, as an impatient person, was difficult. I did however respect that the Covid situation was not to be dismissed and I hoped we'd be starting treatment in a couple of months, when things were better. Looking back, I feel very naïve for expecting to have started treatment in the spring, but I'm proud of myself for overcoming the uncertainty and staying strong.

As many women will remember, as a result of the pandemic and government advice, the HFEA suspended fertility treatment in Q2 2020, and clinics all around the country were forced to stop treatment. It was incredibly heartbreaking but was the right decision to protect everyone. Those months of waiting to start fertility treatment were hard, and my husband and I had no other option but to be patient.

It was during these months, I started to discover the Instagram community of women on their infertility journeys, including those with endometriosis. I discovered the IVF warriors who were documenting their journeys and connecting with this incredible community of strong women, enduring the odds in their pursuit to have their miracle babies. Had I not decided to start my own Instagram account, I wouldn't have connected with so many of the admirable women I speak to today, as we navigate our difficult journeys together in the hope for a happy ending.

Whilst I was comfortable sharing intimate details of my journey, I decided to make the account anonymous, purely to protect my personal life and most importantly my profession, given the incestuous nature of the industry both my husband and I work in. I was relieved that many other accounts I discovered were also anonymous and in a way, it allowed me to be more open about my experiences and feelings without worrying if anyone knew me. Even today, only a handful of the women I've connected with know my name or even what I look like, but I hope one day I will have the confidence and desire to share more about my life and stand proud to be part of this community, with my identity public.

Whilst waiting for the fertility treatment to resume, I had time to educate myself on the IVF process itself, which in a weird way, was a positive take on a frustrating situation that was outside of my control. I'll be honest and say that at times, I really struggled to accept that time was passing us by and we were no closer to starting treatment. Of course, during this time we tried naturally and I hoped we'd be one of those couples who conceived just before starting fertility treatment... unfortunately, we weren't one of those couples. I also found it difficult to relax during this period, which probably didn't help, and with the growing restrictions associated with the pandemic, other usual distractions such as taking holidays or socialising with friends and family were impacted, which for me, made the whole infertility struggle even more 'real' as there weren't any ways to stop thinking about it.

When the HFEA granted authority for certain fertility clinics to recommence treatment, I remember checking their website daily to see if our clinic had been announced on the list. The day I saw our clinic listed, I instantly called them in delight, expecting that this would mean our treatment would resume shortly. Unfortunately though, I was informed that as a result of the closure, there was a long waiting list of women who'd been impacted prior to me starting my treatment (which must have been extremely difficult for them). I was told we would just have to wait a while longer, until we were closer to the front of the queue, so to speak. This was difficult because around this time, I had also been made redundant and I felt like the universe was really testing me. I remained resilient and despite a few wobbles, I got through it and found another job, while continuing to wait to hear from our clinic about when treatment could begin.

Roughly five months after we'd been told IVF was

our best option, we finally got the call, and we had our virtual nurse consultation to sign consent forms. My husband and I were excited and nervous at the same time. During this call, we were given approximate dates of when treatment would begin based on my menstrual cycle. It was a really surreal moment as we entered a new chapter of an unknown experience.

As a married couple, infertility has definitely been hard on us but we have grown so much closer, which I never thought was possible. While I would've preferred not to have waited those five months to start the treatment, looking back it was a blessing in disguise, as it gave me the time to research the process and connect with women via my Instagram, which I really think helped me prepare emotionally and physically. I'm very much a planner in life, so knowing we now had a plan in place gave me an incredible sense of relief and direction. It really enabled me to think much more positively and gave me a new sense of hope.

Prior to starting TTC, after we got married I had started taking prenatal supplements with folic acid and vitamin D. In the months I waited to start IVF, I discovered some other supplements such as Coq10, that could benefit egg quality – which I'd sadly learnt can be impacted by endometriosis. I also introduced more things into my diet including avocado, eggs and pomegranate juice, and was heavily influenced by the many women in the TTC community who were sharing their diet and recipe tips.

For me, the most daunting part of starting IVF was the prospect of the daily injections. I've never been a fan of needles, I mean, who is? I've had some horrible experiences when having blood tests and feeling faint, but in hindsight, the feelings of nausea and feeling faint could have been symptoms of my endometriosis prior to being diagnosed. Either way, I knew that for me the injections would probably be the hardest part. I was actually very wrong.

Following our collection of the drugs, and a face-to-face nurse consultation including a demonstration of how to administer the injections, I actually found the self-injecting part really straightforward. Prior to starting the injections, I also had a baseline scan during my menstrual cycle, to check there were no concerns with my ovaries, uterus or pelvic organs before the treatment commenced. I was told I'd be put on a 'long protocol', which essentially includes a period of down regulation where the medication I was injecting, Buserelin, would switch off my ovaries and stop follicles producing eggs. Then, I would start the stimulation drug (Gonal F®) to hyper stimulate my follicles to grow lots of eggs, ready for collection.

As I've mentioned previously, I really believe the thought of the unknown is often far worse than the reality of the situation. This was definitely my experience of the injections involved with IVF, and the hardest part of the whole experience for both my husband and I, was the emotional aspect – especially after the egg collection procedure. I actually look back at those first weeks of daily injections with fond memories, as fortunately my husband and I were both working from home at the time, and we adopted a strict routine to ensure the injections were administered at the same time every morning. I would also have a 'shot' of pomegranate juice after each injection, which was delicious!

During the down regulation stage, I had a number of transvaginal scans with 'Wanda' at the clinic – all conveniently scheduled prior to work in order to be discreet. These confirmed that my body was responding well to the drugs. Every scan made me feel really positive as I worked my way through an experience that I never thought I'd have to endure. Looking back, the period between starting down regulation and administering the 'trigger' shot of Ovitrelle® (36 hours prior to egg collection) felt really quick, when in reality it was about three to four weeks.

At that stage, all I was thinking about was how many eggs would be retrieved, and the fear again of having to have a general anaesthetic. I reminded myself that I'd had one previously for my laparoscopy and I woke up to tell the tale, so my self-talk really helped keep me feeling strong. Naturally, with the growing Instagram accounts I was discovering who shared details of their IVF journeys, I was worried that my egg collection numbers wouldn't compare. I've come to realise through this journey though that everyone's experiences really are different and whilst there are key characteristics that are the same (such as the egg collection and transfer procedures), the moments in between can really vary – including how women respond to the drugs and the number of eggs retrieved.

I remember hoping for 10 eggs, as during the scans there were at least 10 follicles of good size. You can imagine our delight after the egg collection, when the embryologist told us we had 14 eggs ready to be fertilised. Even the general anaesthetic injection was fine and I didn't bother with the numbing cream, so was very proud of myself… despite feeling mortified about the physical position I was put in for the collection itself, with my legs very spread! When I woke up in the hospital bed afterwards, I had absolutely no recollection of the procedure nor did I have any pain or discomfort, which was a relief. I do realise some women's experiences aren't like this though and having read some stories both prior to and after my procedure, my heart really goes out to those who've had traumatic experiences. As I said before, every journey is different and no two experiences are the same. I only wish that all experiences in this horrible journey could be positive.

I mentioned earlier that the hardest part of the journey is the emotional side. The days following the egg collection were seriously difficult and my husband and I were required to remain patient whilst we awaited phone calls from the clinic with updates on the fertilisation rates of my 14 eggs. Unfortunately, the day after the collection we were informed that of the 14 collected eggs, only five had fertilised into embryos. We had no reason to have opted to have ICSI because my husband's semen analysis showed good results, so we still to this day don't understand why less than 50% fertilised, when clinics usually expect to see at least a 70% fertilisation rate.

Honestly, we weren't expecting such a drop in numbers, so this news did come as quite a shock. Unsurprisingly, this made us feel anxious and damaged our sense of hope. We tried to remain positive for the five fertilised eggs and hoped that one of those would become our baby. 'It only takes one' was our mantra for the days that followed. Most clinics will provide you with an update on your embryos on day 3, and we couldn't wait for the call to find out how our embryos were doing. Unfortunately, we were informed that only three were growing well, and by day 5 (the day of my transfer), we were told that one wasn't growing as quickly and wasn't able to be frozen, and the remaining two were 'early blastocysts' and also weren't able to be frozen as they hadn't reached the optimum levels required. That meant only two were viable for embryo transfer.

We were asked to consider whether we'd like to transfer the two early blastocysts, or just one, in the knowledge that this would mean the other would be destroyed. My husband and I were completely on the same page and we agreed to transfer both. We had always considered the possibility of twins, having heard they can come from IVF treatment, and we understood the risk that both embryos could implant but were comfortable with our decision. I remember we were told that the one remaining embryo may 'speed up' its growth by day 6, so they agreed to leave it for a further day to see if it could reach blastocyst stage and be frozen.

The transfer procedure itself feels like a smear test and it was over very quickly. I was sad my husband couldn't be there with me, but I knew he was waiting eagerly outside in the clinic car park. Following the procedure, in true IVF tradition, we ventured to McDonald's® for takeaway fries – which are said to carry 'luck' within the TTC community once you become PUPO. I also snacked on pineapple for the rest of the day and rested with lots of nice TV.

Fortunately, the transfer was on a Saturday so I didn't need to take any time off work, which was wonderful. This day was also positive because we received the news that our one remaining embryo had caught up and was suitable to freeze for a future round, if we needed it. I couldn't believe it. The one goal we'd had all along was to have embryos to freeze (as well as a successful pregnancy, of course), as having an FET would be less intensive, instead of undergoing a full IVF cycle from scratch including egg collection. Whilst we were disappointed not to have more than one embryo frozen, we were grateful for this one as I know of so many women who sadly don't end up with any to freeze. I've certainly learnt throughout this process that nothing is guaranteed and you cannot control how your body will react or respond. You just have to put your trust in the process and hope that things will all go to plan.

Following embryo transfer, the hardest part of the process emotionally began. The dreaded two-week wait. This period of time is tough for any woman on her journey to conceive, with or without having had fertility treatment, but I do feel that it's much harder when you've gone through so much to even get to that point, let alone what the result may then be. I was also taking two Cyclogest® pessaries daily, which I fortunately didn't find too bad. Due to the ongoing pandemic, we weren't able to physically do much over the two weeks, other than go for nice walks to keep us distracted.

About a week after the transfer itself, I noticed spotting, just like I usually experience prior to a period and I naturally expected the worst. I felt horrifically low. I'd convinced myself that it just hadn't worked but was supported by women in the IVF community, who advised me about 'implantation bleeding'. This, of course, prompted me to research further and give myself peace of mind that the spotting might just be that, and it wasn't a sign of my period or that our two beautiful embryos hadn't made it.

The spotting fortunately settled within about three days and I started to wonder if it could've been a sign of success, however a couple of days before 'official test day', I started to bleed light pink. I instantly thought it was over and took a pregnancy test to confirm my fears. To my utter shock, the test was positive with a faint line. My husband and I just couldn't believe it. This was the first ever positive pregnancy result we'd seen in our years of trying, and it just felt incredibly surreal and exciting. We were pregnant and something in me shifted. I felt amazing. We both knew it was very early days, but I will never forget that feeling in my belly of experiencing a positive pregnancy test, and I hope I get to experience it again one day.

Within the weeks that followed, we shared the news with our closest friends and family who knew we were having treatment and they were overjoyed for us. However, at six weeks pregnant, I began to experience light spotting again. The clinic recommended that I increase my daily progesterone pessaries from twice a day to three times a day. I remember being told that if it remained a light spotting that things should be fine, but I think I already knew in my gut that this wasn't a good sign. I remember a few days of spotting later, when it then turned to a heavy bleed, texting my mum and telling her that I expected I was losing the pregnancy.

I don't think I've ever felt more broken than during those days. We sadly miscarried our two beautiful embryos at six weeks pregnant, which was confirmed during a transvaginal scan at our clinic a few days after the heavy bleeding had stopped. There was a glimmer of hope that there may be something there, but I think sometimes you just know. My husband, as always, was my complete rock, as were our friends and family. We had kept the whole process private from our employers and therefore we didn't share our sad news with them and tried to carry on as 'normal', despite the pain we were both enduring.

This was especially difficult in the build up to Christmas, as Covid restrictions increased, meaning we were unable to physically see or hug anyone when that's all we needed most. This, coupled with the expected Christmas pregnancy announcements on social media, made it exceptionally difficult to find the strength to remain hopeful that our time would come. I found myself submerged in motivational quotes and success stories wherever I could find them online, to keep me positive and hopeful for the future.

I will never forget how strong we were to get through that time and I feel blessed to have had the support we experienced from those we'd told. We shall always feel fortunate that our first round of IVF worked, and we experienced our first positive pregnancy test, but we will always wonder who those embryos would've become and what our world would have been like had we ended up with twins in our lives. We decided not to give them names, as I know some people who share this grief choose to do, which is such a personal decision to make.

For us, whilst we will always remember those embryos and that they were part of us, we feel strangely grateful that it was an early miscarriage and not at a later stage – like my poor parents had endured at 18 weeks. I also didn't need any further medical intervention, which was a relief. Regardless of the timing of the miscarriage, it was hard, but we dusted ourselves off and carried on. That's resilience for you, and I am amazed that my husband and I found that inner strength to keep going. We utilised the counselling service that was part of our IVF package and spoke openly with a counsellor about how we were feeling, which was a really positive and valuable experience to help us make sense of the situation and find coping mechanisms to manage our emotions.

As I mentioned, I am a planner, and whilst we were

still grieving the miscarriage, we agreed that we should have a plan in place for our one remaining frozen embryo, to give us something to focus on. A few weeks after the miscarriage, we scheduled another consultation with our clinic to plan a frozen embryo transfer. Fortunately, things moved very quickly and before I knew it, the drugs were purchased and I was having my baseline scan again. During this scan however, the nurse identified what she believed to be a suspected polyp. My heart and stomach sank as it felt like another obstacle in an already challenging journey. I was told to return to the clinic the following day for a further scan to check, with the knowledge that if it was still there, we'd have to stop our fertility treatment and have the polyp removed via a hysteroscopy. Being the impatient person that I am, I was so upset with the prospect of a delay.

At the scan the following day however, no such polyp was located and I felt an incredible sense of relief that our FET could proceed. I actually found the drugs in preparation for transfer incredibly easy compared to the fresh IVF cycle, as there wasn't a down regulation phase and it felt more natural. I was required to take tablets four times a day (containing oestrogen) and I had scans to check the thickness of my uterus lining, to ensure it was suitable for the transfer to increase the chance of the embryo implanting. It is such a fascinating and clever process when you consider all the steps that need to be taken to maximise your chances of becoming pregnant, and it often blows my mind that IVF even exists.

After the transfer was scheduled, the next hurdle was whether the frozen embryo would survive the thawing process on transfer day. I remember being extremely anxious and restless the night before and morning of the transfer, waiting for the call to confirm if the transfer would go ahead. My husband was confident that all would be fine (and yes, he was in fact right!). Despite being told that the thawing process is very safe and that 95% of embryos survive the thaw, I knew of several women in the TTC community who had sadly lost their embryos at this stage, so my imagination was uncontrollable – especially as this was our last and only embryo from our fresh IVF cycle. If this didn't work, we would have to start from scratch. I knew it wasn't our 'last chance' but it felt that way at times.

I could've cried with happiness when the embryologist called (after I'd called them, being the impatient person that I am!) to confirm that our 4BB grade embryo had survived the thaw and they would look forward to seeing me for the transfer in the few hours that followed. I would recommend anyone having a transfer, where it falls on a weekday, to try and have the full day off work if you can. I am so glad that I did, as whilst the procedure isn't very long, it really does consume you emotionally. I really don't think that I would've been able to detach myself from 'work mode' to embrace the experience had I not taken the full day.

I have to be honest and say that, this time, the transfer wasn't as quick as the previous experience. It also wasn't as comfortable unfortunately, because it just seemed to take forever. I did get to see the embryo on a screen though, which I didn't get to experience before due to a different person doing the transfer, so that was one positive and it was a very magical moment. I would still describe the procedure as similar to a smear test, however this particular transfer felt like a really long smear test. Of course, I would do it all over again (and I know now, writing this, that I will have to) but it wasn't as pleasant as I'd hoped. I think also that my emotions at the time didn't help the situation. I knew at that moment it was our last embryo, and it was another reminder that my body cannot do what I thought it would be able to do and become pregnant naturally, as a biological woman. I just wanted the procedure over and done with.

Sadly, following the second transfer and the dreaded two-week wait, we got a BFN result. We were both incredibly disappointed as we knew that our first IVF cycle had officially reached its conclusion, and we had no more frozen embryos left to transfer. I personally felt like my grief was amplified this time, as I felt sadness for the negative result, but also for the loss of my pregnancy just a couple of months prior. I maintained my resilience, together with my husband, and fortunately the negative result came on a Friday evening, so we had the weekend to process and mourn the situation, whilst indulging in lots of self-care and without having to 'fake it' at work for a few days.

Fortunately, working from home as a result of the pandemic meant that I was close to my husband when I needed him during the working day, and I didn't have to 'keep face' as I would've done in an office setting. The best way to describe that feeling was emptiness, because I knew the negative result meant that we would have to start everything all over again. During this time, our consultant also left our clinic due to changes in the company and this only added to my already increasing anxiety. It was difficult given there were a lot of 'endings' taking place. By speaking about how I was feeling to my mum and my husband, it really helped me to think rationally and within a matter of weeks, following our negative result, we were back at our clinic, meeting with a new consultant to agree our next steps.

At this moment, writing my story, my husband and I are soon to be starting a new fresh cycle. With ICSI instead of IVF this time and on a short protocol, in the hope that this will increase our fertilisation rates following the next egg collection, and hopefully the eggs collected will be of a higher quality. I am feeling extremely nervous about what is yet to come, but I will continue to remind myself that I can do this, despite the physical and emotional burden. My husband and I are a team and we have an incredible support network. We aren't ready to give up on our dream to become parents and this is another stepping stone and chapter in our story, which hopefully will reach a happy ending. The biggest advice I would give to anyone going through a similar journey is to seek support and speak to your loved ones where you feel it will help you. You are not alone and infertility is not your fault, so please try not to punish yourself for things that you cannot control or question your self-worth. I am guilty of this some days, but I have learnt over the last two years to improve my 'negative self-talk' and this has helped me find the strength and resilience to keep going. I would also really recommend utilising the counselling services that your clinic offer (which is usually a feature of any treatment package), as it really helped us during our first IVF cycle.

Closing comments

We often refer to many elements of our lives as being on a journey. Life in itself is a journey if you think about it deeply, and every journey is full of obstacles and crossroads that give our lives meaning and direction. With infertility, the best way to describe this journey (which helps me) is to literally imagine a pathway. No one can see the end of the pathway, but you can see along the way that there are a series of junctions, just like you'd take if you were physically walking on this path. In this scenario, similar to how we navigate our infertility journeys, there is no map to tell us what route we should take, only offered guidance on what routes are available to consider. We therefore just have to trust the journey and sometimes discover new routes and enter the unknown to keep us moving forward.

These junctions in the pathway represent new opportunities, that we can choose whether or not to explore further. These also represent those moments where unexpected events happen – for example, if during your fertility treatment you don't respond as expected to the drugs or the fertilisation rate is below average. These are all outside of your control but all you can do is keep going on your journey, finding new junctions and making new decisions, until you hopefully reach your destination, and your end goal and purpose of your journey, to meet your baby.

I'd like to conclude my story by emphasising the importance of supporting one another and most importantly, that we have 'hope'. For me, hope is one of the most powerful words used in our lives, and especially within the infertility community. It's that feeling of expectation and desire for a particular thing to happen, and in that feeling it promotes an optimistic state of mind. As a verb, hope is also defined as 'expect with confidence' and 'to cherish a desire with anticipation'. We may not have reached our desired destination, and we may not even be close to the end of our destined pathway, but as long as we maintain hope,

I know one way or another, my husband and I will get there and someone, one day, will call us 'Mummy' and 'Daddy' and this journey will feel completely worth it.

Chosen charity

Our charity is Oscar's Wish Foundation: www.oscarswishfoundation.co.uk

They offer comfort and support to parents, family, friends and siblings who have experienced the devastating loss of a precious baby before, during or shortly after birth.

Our charities

- Fertility Network UK:
  fertilitynetworkuk.org

- Miscarriage Association:
  www.miscarriageassociation.org.uk

- Resolve:
  resolve.org

- The Chris Aked Foundation:
  www.chrisakedfoundation.co.uk

- The Survivors Trust:
  www.thesurvivorstrust.org/pbpaftercsa

- Donor Conception Network:
  www.dcnetwork.org

- CoppaFeel!:
  coppafeel.org

- Future Dreams:
  futuredreams.org.uk

- Pink Elephants:
  www.pinkelephants.org.au

- The Bumpy Foundation:
  www.facebook.com/thebumpyfoundation

- Tommy's:
  www.tommys.org

- Tiny Life:
  www.tinylife.org.uk

- Adapt Domestic Abuse Services:
  adaptservices.ie

- The Broken Brown Egg:
  thebrokenbrownegg.org

- The Ectopic Pregnancy Trust:
  ectopic.org.uk

- Oscar's Wish Foundation:
  www.oscarswishfoundation.co.uk

Thank you...

For reading our stories and for helping us
raise money for our chosen charities.

We hope our journeys will offer you support,
hope and the knowledge that you are not alone.

Connect with us on Instagram:
@weareoneineight

Printed in Great Britain
by Amazon